Metabolic Confusion Diet Cookbook For Endomorphs Women

The Science-Backed Guide to Sustainable Weight Loss, Fat Burning, and Metabolism Boosting with Delicious, No-Stress Recipes | Full Color Pictures & 28-Day Meal Plan Included to Live a Vibrant Life

TIMOTHY A. GWIN

Copyright Page

TABLE OF CONTENTS

Introduction

- Understanding the Endomorph Body Type 6
- Characteristic of Endomorphs 6

The Science behind Metabolic Confusion

- What is an Metabolic Confusion? 8
- Understanding Metabolism and Hormones 9

Benefits of the Metabolic Confusion Diet

- Real-Life Benefits 10

Setting Your Goals

- Understanding your WHY 11

Essential Kitchen Tools

- Must Have Appliances 12

Stocking Your Pantry

- Essential Ingredients 13
- Creating Balanced Meal Plans 14
- Grocery Shopping Tips 15

- **Food to Include & Avoid For Endomorphs** 16

Exercise and Lifestyle Tips 22

- Importance of Physical Activity

Effective Workouts For Endomorph Women   23

- Stress Management Techniques   24
- Importance of Sleep   25

- **Success Stories and Testimonials**   26
- **Tips from Successful Dieters**   27
- **Motivational Stories**   28
- **28-Day Meal Plan**   30

RECIPES

- Avocado and Smoked Salmon Toast   34
- Greek Yogurt Parfait   35
- Berry Blast Quinoa Breakfast Bowl   36
- Tropical Paradise Quinoa Breakfast Bowl   37
- Peanut Butter Banana Smoothie   38
- Oatmeal with Nuts and Berries   39
- Turkey and Cheese Omelette   40

- Low-Calories Tofu Scramble   41
- Grilled Chicken and Avocado Salad   42
- Turkey and Quinoa Stuffed Peppers   43
- Beef and Broccoli Stir-Fry   44
- Salmon and Avocado Sushi Bowl   45
- Mediterranean Tuna and White Bean Salad   46
- Avocado Tuna and White Bean Salad   47
- Turkey Lettuce Wraps   48

- Spicy veggie and Hummus Wrap — 50
- Chickpea and Avocado Salad Sandwich — 51
- Zucchini Noodles with Pesto — 52
- Baked Sweet Potato Fries — 53
- Chicken and Pesto Pasta — 54
- Shrimp and Veggie Stir-Fry — 55
- Turkey Meatballs — 56
- Baked Cod with Roasted Veggies — 57
- Hard Boiled Eggs — 58
- Cucumber Slices with Tzatziki — 59
- Zoodle Pad Thai — 60
- Cauliflower Fried Rice — 62
- Grilled Portobello Mushrooms — 64
- Air Popped Popcorn — 66
- Chicken and Veggie kebabs — 67
- Salmon and Spinach Salad — 68
- **Importance of Consistency** — 70
- **Balancing Cardio & Strength Training** — 71
- **List of Exercises** — 72
- **Tips for success** — 74

WELCOME TO THE METABOLIC CONFUSION DIET

This book is designed to guide you through the intricacies of the metabolic confusion diet, a unique approach to weight loss and health optimization that caters specifically to the needs of endomorph women. Whether you're new to the concept or have some experience, this cookbook aims to provide you with the knowledge, tools, and delicious recipes needed to achieve your health and fitness goals.

UNDERSTANDING THE ENDOMORPH BODY TYPE

Endomorphs are characterized by a higher percentage of body fat, a wider waist, and a tendency to gain weight easily, especially in the lower body. Metabolism tends to be slower in endomorphs, making weight loss more challenging compared to other body types. However, with the right approach, endomorphs can achieve significant improvements in their body composition and overall health.

Characteristics of Endomorphs:
- **Higher Body Fat Percentage:** Endomorphs naturally carry more body fat.
- **Slower Metabolism:** Weight gain occurs more easily due to a slower metabolic rate.
- **Carbohydrate Sensitivity:** Endomorphs often respond better to lower-carb diets.

THE SCIENCE BEHIND METABOLIC CONFUSION

- **What is Metabolic Confusion?**

Metabolic confusion, also known as calorie shifting, is a dietary strategy designed to prevent the body from adapting to a constant caloric intake. The fundamental principle involves varying daily calorie consumption to "confuse" the metabolism, keeping it active and efficient. By alternating between high-calorie and low-calorie days, the body avoids entering a plateau phase, which is a common challenge in traditional dieting.

- **How It Works**

Metabolic confusion leverages the body's natural metabolic responses to varying calorie intakes. When calories are consistently reduced, the body adapts by lowering the metabolic rate to conserve energy. This adaptation can slow weight loss and lead to plateaus. However, by varying caloric intake, the body remains in a state of heightened metabolic activity, promoting continued fat loss and preventing metabolic slowdown.

Benefits of Metabolic Confusion

- **Sustained Weight Loss:** By preventing metabolic adaptation, metabolic confusion supports continuous weight loss.
- **Reduced Hunger and Cravings:** Varying calorie intake can help manage hunger and reduce cravings, making it easier to stick to the diet.
- **Increased Energy Levels:** The periodic increase in calories can boost energy levels and improve workout performance.
- **Flexibility and Variety:** This approach allows for a more varied diet, making it easier to adhere to over the long term.

- **The Role of Macronutrients**

Macronutrients—proteins, fats, and carbohydrates—are essential components of our diet. Understanding how they impact metabolism is crucial for implementing a metabolic confusion diet effectively.

- **Proteins:** Essential for muscle repair and growth, proteins have a high thermic effect, meaning the body burns more calories digesting them. Including high-protein foods can enhance metabolic rate.
- **Fats:** Healthy fats provide a long-lasting source of energy and are essential for hormone production. Incorporating good fats ensures balanced energy levels and supports metabolic health.
- **Carbohydrates:** Carbs are the body's primary energy source. Strategic consumption of carbs, especially complex carbohydrates, provides sustained energy and prevents insulin spikes.

- **Understanding Metabolism and Hormones**

Metabolism encompasses all the chemical reactions in the body that convert food into energy. Several hormones play a pivotal role in regulating metabolism:

- **Insulin:** Regulates blood sugar levels and influences fat storage. Managing insulin through balanced meals is crucial.
- **Leptin and Ghrelin:** These hormones regulate hunger and satiety. Leptin decreases appetite, while ghrelin stimulates it. Calorie variation can help maintain healthy levels of these hormones.
- **Cortisol:** Known as the stress hormone, elevated cortisol levels can lead to weight gain, particularly around the abdomen. Managing stress is essential for maintaining a healthy metabolism.

BENEFITS OF THE METABOLIC CONFUSION DIET FOR ENDOMORPH WOMEN

Tailoring the Diet for Endomorph Women

- **Caloric Cycling:** Alternating between high and low-calorie days helps keep the metabolism active, promoting fat loss without the body adapting to a constant caloric intake.
- **Macronutrient Balance:** Emphasizing proteins and healthy fats while managing carbohydrate intake can support sustained energy and reduce fat storage.
- **Hormonal Balance:** The diet's structure helps regulate key hormones, reducing hunger and preventing stress-related weight gain.

Real-Life Benefits

- **Enhanced Fat Loss**: By preventing metabolic slowdown, endomorph women can experience more consistent and significant fat loss.
- **Improved Energy Levels**: The periodic increase in calories helps maintain energy levels, making it easier to stay active and exercise regularly.
- **Better Adherence**: The flexibility and variety of the diet make it more sustainable and enjoyable, reducing the likelihood of giving up.

The metabolic confusion diet offers a scientifically-backed approach to weight loss, particularly beneficial for endomorph women. By understanding the principles of metabolic confusion, the role of macronutrients, and the hormonal influences on metabolism, individuals can tailor their diet to achieve optimal results. The benefits of this diet extend beyond weight loss, promoting overall metabolic health, energy balance, and long-term adherence.

SETTING YOUR GOALS

UNDERSTANDING YOUR WHY

Before embarking on the Metabolic Confusion Diet, it's crucial to understand your motivation. Ask yourself:

- **Why do you want to follow this diet?**
- **What are your long-term health and fitness goals?**
- **How will achieving these goals improve your life?**

Defining Clear Objectives

Set specific, measurable, achievable, relevant, and time-bound (SMART) goals. Examples include:

- Lose 10 pounds in three months
- Reduce body fat percentage by 5% in six months
- Increase daily energy levels and reduce fatigue

Tracking Progress

Monitoring your progress helps keep you motivated and on track. Consider:

- Weekly weigh-ins
- Measuring body fat percentage
- Taking progress photos
- Keeping a food and exercise journal

Regular Check-Ins

Schedule regular check-ins to review your progress:

- Weekly: Review weight, measurements, and food logs
- Monthly: Assess overall progress and make necessary adjustments
- Quarterly: Evaluate long-term goals and achievements

ESSENTIAL KITCHEN TOOLS

MUST-HAVE APPLIANCES

Invest in essential kitchen appliances to streamline meal prep:

- **Blender:** For smoothies and purees
- **Food Processor:** For chopping and mixing
- **Slow Cooker:** For easy, hands-off cooking
- **Instant Pot:** For versatile, quick meals
- **Air Fryer:** For healthier frying options

UTENSILS AND GADGETS

Equip your kitchen with the right utensils and gadgets:

- **Sharp Knives:** For efficient chopping
- **Cutting Boards:** Separate ones for meat and vegetables
- **Measuring Cups and Spoons:** For accurate portioning
- **Mixing Bowls:** Various sizes for different tasks
- **Non-Stick Cookware:** For easy cooking and cleaning

STORAGE SOLUTIONS

Organize your kitchen with proper storage solutions:

- **Glass Containers:** For meal prep and storage
- **Mason Jars:** For smoothies and dry goods
- **Freezer Bags:** For storing prepped ingredients
- **Spice Rack:** For easy access to seasonings
- **Label Maker:** For identifying stored items

STOCKING YOUR PANTRY

ESSENTIAL INGREDIENTS

Stock your pantry with essential ingredients for the Metabolic Confusion Diet:

- **Proteins**: Chicken, turkey, lean beef, tofu, tempeh
- **Carbohydrates**: Quinoa, brown rice, sweet potatoes, whole grain pasta
- **Healthy Fats:** Olive oil, avocado, nuts, seeds
- **Vegetables:** Leafy greens, bell peppers, broccoli, zucchini
- **Fruits:** Berries, apples, bananas, citrus fruits

SPICES AND SEASONINGS

Enhance your meals with a variety of spices and seasonings:

- **Herbs:** Basil, cilantro, parsley, rosemary
- **Spices:** Cumin, turmeric, paprika, cinnamon
- **Condiments**: Soy sauce, hot sauce, mustard, balsamic vinegar
- **Flavorings:** Garlic, ginger, lemon, lime

MEAL PREP STAPLES

Keep these staples on hand for quick meal prep:

- **Broths:** Chicken, beef, and vegetable
- **Canned Goods:** Beans, tomatoes, tuna, salmon
- **Frozen Vegetables:** Spinach, peas, mixed vegetables
- **Whole Grains:** Oats, barley, farro
- **Nut Butters:** Almond, peanut, cashew

CREATING BALANCED MEAL PLANS

Macronutrient Balance

Ensure each meal contains a balance of macronutrients:

- **Proteins:** Aim for a source of lean protein in every meal
- **Carbohydrates:** Include complex carbohydrates for sustained energy
- **Fats:** Incorporate healthy fats for satiety and flavor

Portion Control

Use portion control techniques to avoid overeating:

- **Hand Method:** Use your hand to estimate portion sizes (e.g., palm-sized portion of protein, fist-sized portion of vegetables)
- **Plate Method:** Fill half your plate with vegetables, one-quarter with protein, and one-quarter with carbohydrates
- **Weighing and Measuring:** Use kitchen scales and measuring cups for accuracy

Meal Timing

Distribute your meals throughout the day to maintain energy levels:

- **Breakfast:** Within an hour of waking
- **Lunch:** Midday to refuel
- **Dinner:** Early evening to prevent late-night snacking
- **Snacks:** As needed between meals

GROCERY SHOPPING TIPS

Planning Ahead

Create a grocery list based on your meal plan:

- **Weekly Planning:** Plan meals for the week and make a detailed list
- **Bulk Buying:** Purchase non-perishable items in bulk to save money
- **Seasonal Shopping:** Choose seasonal produce for freshness and cost savings

Smart Shopping Strategies

Use these strategies to shop efficiently:

- **Stick to the List:** Avoid impulse buys by sticking to your list
- **Shop the Perimeter:** Focus on the store's perimeter where fresh produce, meats, and dairy are located
- **Read Labels:** Check labels for added sugars, unhealthy fats, and sodium

Budget-Friendly Tips

Save money while maintaining a healthy diet:

- **Buy Generic:** Opt for store brands when possible
- **Use Coupons:** Look for discounts and coupons on healthy items
- **Frozen Options:** Choose frozen fruits and vegetables when fresh ones are too expensive

FOODS TO INCLUDE AND AVOID FOR ENDOMORPHS

Endomorphs are characterized by a higher propensity to store fat, a rounder body shape, and a slower metabolism. People with this body type often find it challenging to lose weight and may gain weight easily if their diet is not well- managed.

BEST FOODS FOR ENDOMORPHS

To manage their weight and optimize their health, endomorphs should focus on a diet that is balanced but slightly skewed towards certain macronutrients.

Proteins:

- **Lean Meats:** Chicken breast, turkey, and lean cuts of beef or pork provide high-quality protein without excessive fat.
- **Fish:** Particularly fatty fish like salmon, mackerel, and sardines, which are rich in omega-3 fatty acids that can help reduce inflammation and improve metabolism.
- **Eggs:** A great source of protein and essential nutrients, eggs can be included in various meals.
- **Legumes:** Beans, lentils, and chickpeas offer both protein and fiber, helping with satiety and digestive health.

Vegetables:

- **Leafy Greens:** Spinach, kale, and Swiss chard are low in calories and high in essential vitamins and minerals.
- **Cruciferous Vegetables:** Broccoli, cauliflower, and Brussels sprouts are nutrient-dense and support detoxification processes.
- **Colorful Veggies:** Peppers, carrots, and tomatoes provide a variety of vitamins and antioxidants.

Fruits:

- **Berries:** Blueberries, strawberries, and raspberries are low in sugar and high in fiber and antioxidants.
- **Citrus Fruits:** Oranges, lemons, and grapefruits are good sources of vitamin C and fiber.
- **Apples and Pears:** High in fiber, these fruits can help with fullness and provide steady energy.

Whole Grains:

- **Quinoa:** A high-protein grain that is also gluten-free and packed with nutrients.
- **Brown Rice:** Provides sustained energy and fiber, supporting digestive health.
- **Oats:** Great for breakfast, oats are high in soluble fiber, which helps control blood sugar levels.

Healthy Fats:

- **Avocados:** Rich in monounsaturated fats and fiber, avocados support heart health and satiety.
- **Nuts and Seeds:** Almonds, chia seeds, and flaxseeds provide healthy fats, fiber, and protein.
- **Olive Oil:** A staple of the Mediterranean diet, olive oil is rich in heart-healthy monounsaturated fats.

Dairy:

- **Low-Fat Yogurt:** Offers protein and probiotics, beneficial for gut health.
- **Cottage Cheese:** High in protein and low in fat, it's a versatile dairy option.
- **Milk:** Preferably low-fat or skim, milk provides essential nutrients like calcium and vitamin D.

FOODS TO MINIMIZE OR AVOID

Endomorphs should minimize or avoid foods that can contribute to fat storage and metabolic slowdowns.

Refined Carbohydrates:

- **White Bread and Pastries:** These offer little nutritional value and can spike blood sugar levels.
- **Sugary Cereals:** Often high in added sugars and low in fiber, they can lead to energy crashes.
- **White Pasta and Rice:** Opt for whole grain versions to get more fiber and nutrients.

Sugary Foods and Drinks:

- **Soda and Sweetened Beverages:** High in empty calories and sugars, they can lead to weight gain and metabolic issues.
- **Candy and Sweets:** These provide excessive sugar without any nutritional benefits.
- **Desserts:** Cakes, cookies, and ice cream should be occasional treats due to their high sugar and fat content.

Processed Foods:

- **Processed Meats:** Sausages, hot dogs, and deli meats often contain high levels of unhealthy fats and sodium.
- **Ready-to-Eat Meals:** These can be high in unhealthy fats, sugars, and sodium.
- **Snack Foods:** Chips, crackers, and similar snacks usually contain refined carbs and unhealthy fats.

High-Fat Foods:

- **Fried Foods:** French fries, fried chicken, and other deep-fried items can add excessive calories and unhealthy fats.
- **High-Fat Dairy:** Full-fat cheese, cream, and butter should be limited due to their high saturated fat content.
- **Certain Oils:** Avoid trans fats and limit saturated fats, opting for healthier oils like olive or avocado oil instead.

UNDERSTANDING FOOD LABELS

Reading and understanding food labels can help endomorphs make healthier choices and avoid foods that may hinder their weight management goals.

Serving Size:

- Always check the serving size first. Many packaged foods contain multiple servings, and consuming more than the serving size listed will increase the intake of all listed nutrients, including calories, fats, and sugars.

Calories:

- Pay attention to the number of calories per serving and how they fit into your daily caloric needs.

Macronutrients:

- Total Fat: Look for the types of fat included. Aim for foods low in saturated and trans fats.
- Carbohydrates: Focus on the amount of dietary fiber and sugars. Higher fiber is better, and lower added sugars are preferable.
- Protein: A higher protein content can help with satiety and muscle maintenance.

Micronutrients:

- Check for essential vitamins and minerals like vitamin D, calcium, iron, and potassium. These are often under-consumed nutrients.

Ingredient List:

- Ingredients are listed in descending order by weight. Aim for foods with whole, recognizable ingredients. Avoid products where sugar or unhealthy fats appear high on the list.

Daily Value Percentages:

- These percentages help you understand how a serving of the food contributes to your daily nutrient needs based on a 2,000-calorie diet. Aim for lower percentages of saturated fats, added sugars, and sodium, and higher percentages of fiber, vitamins, and minerals.

For endomorphs, managing diet is crucial to balance metabolism, control weight, and maintain overall health. Focusing on nutrient-dense foods like lean proteins, vegetables, fruits, whole grains, and healthy fats, while minimizing refined carbs, sugary foods, processed items, and unhealthy fats, can make a significant difference. Additionally, understanding and using food labels can guide better food choices, supporting a healthier lifestyle tailored to the endomorph body type.

EXERCISE AND LIFESTYLE TIPS

IMPORTANCE OF PHYSICAL ACTIVITY

Regular physical activity is a crucial component of the Metabolic Confusion Diet for endomorph women. This chapter will delve into why exercise is vital for boosting metabolism, enhancing weight loss, and improving overall health.

Benefits of Physical Activity

- **Increased Metabolic Rate:** Exercise helps increase your metabolic rate, which is essential for endomorphs who typically have a slower metabolism.
- **Muscle Building:** Strength training exercises help build lean muscle mass, which in turn increases the number of calories burned at rest.
- **Fat Loss:** Regular aerobic and anaerobic activities help reduce body fat, especially in stubborn areas common to endomorphs.
- **Improved Insulin Sensitivity:** Exercise improves insulin sensitivity, helping to regulate blood sugar levels and reduce the risk of type 2 diabetes.
- **Enhanced Mood and Energy Levels:** Physical activity releases endorphins, which improve mood and increase energy levels.
- **Cardiovascular Health:** Regular exercise strengthens the heart and improves cardiovascular health.

EFFECTIVE WORKOUTS FOR ENDOMORPH WOMEN

This section will provide detailed guidance on the types of workouts that are most effective for endomorph women. It will include a mix of strength training, cardio, and flexibility exercises designed to maximize metabolic confusion and promote fat loss.

Strength Training

Strength training is particularly beneficial for endomorphs as it helps build muscle and boost metabolism.

- **Resistance Training:** Incorporate exercises like squats, lunges, deadlifts, and bench presses.
- **Circuit Training:** Combine multiple exercises in a circuit format to keep the heart rate up and burn more calories.
- **Bodyweight Exercises:** Push-ups, pull-ups, and bodyweight squats are effective for building strength without needing equipment.

CARDIOVASCULAR EXERCISE

Cardio is essential for burning calories and improving heart health.

- **High-Intensity Interval Training (HIIT):** Short bursts of intense exercise followed by brief rest periods. This can include sprints, jump squats, and burpees.
- **Steady-State Cardio:** Activities like jogging, cycling, and swimming at a moderate pace for an extended period.
- **Low-Impact Cardio:** Walking, elliptical training, and water aerobics are easier on the joints and still effective for burning calories.

FLEXIBILITY AND RECOVERY

Flexibility exercises and proper recovery are crucial for preventing injuries and maintaining a balanced workout routine.

- **Yoga:** Improves flexibility, reduces stress, and enhances overall well-being.
- **Stretching:** Incorporate both dynamic and static stretching to improve range of motion and prevent muscle stiffness.
- **Foam Rolling:** Helps relieve muscle tightness and improve blood flow to the muscles.

STRESS MANAGEMENT TECHNIQUES

Managing stress is a critical aspect of the Metabolic Confusion Diet, as high stress levels can negatively impact metabolism and weight loss efforts.

Mindfulness and Meditation

- **Mindfulness Practices**: Techniques such as deep breathing, body scans, and mindful eating.
- **Meditation**: Guided meditations, mindfulness meditation, and progressive muscle relaxation.

Stress-Reducing Activities

- **Hobbies**: Engaging in activities you enjoy, such as reading, gardening, or crafting.
- **Nature Walks**: Spending time outdoors to relax and reduce stress levels.
- **Social Connections**: Maintaining healthy relationships and seeking support from friends and family.

Sleep and Recovery Tips

Adequate sleep and proper recovery are essential for maintaining a healthy metabolism and overall well-being.

IMPORTANCE OF SLEEP

- **Metabolic Health**: Poor sleep can disrupt hormonal balance and metabolism.
- **Recovery**: Sleep is crucial for muscle recovery and repair after workouts.
- **Mental Health**: Quality sleep improves mood, cognitive function, and stress resilience.

TIPS FOR BETTER SLEEP

- **Sleep Hygiene**: Establish a regular sleep routine, create a comfortable sleep environment, and avoid screens before bedtime.
- **Relaxation Techniques**: Practices such as reading, taking a warm bath, or listening to calming music.
- **Sleep Aids**: Natural supplements like melatonin or herbal teas (consult with a healthcare provider before use).

By incorporating these exercise and lifestyle tips, endomorph women can maximize the benefits of the Metabolic Confusion Diet, achieving their health and fitness goals while maintaining a balanced and fulfilling lifestyle.

SUCCESS STORIES AND TESTIMONIALS

REAL-LIFE TRANSFORMATIONS

Case Study 1: Sarah's Journey

Sarah, a 35-year-old endomorph woman, struggled with weight loss for years despite trying numerous diets. After discovering the Metabolic Confusion Diet, she experienced remarkable changes. Over six months, Sarah lost 30 pounds and significantly improved her energy levels. By alternating between high-calorie and low-calorie days, she found a sustainable way to keep her metabolism active. Sarah's dedication to meal prepping and regular exercise played a crucial role in her success. Her story highlights the effectiveness of metabolic confusion in overcoming weight loss plateaus.

Case Study 2: Emily's Transformation

Emily, a 40-year-old mother of two, faced challenges balancing her busy life with healthy eating. The flexibility of the Metabolic Confusion Diet allowed her to plan meals that fit her family's schedule. Emily lost 25 pounds in five months and gained a newfound confidence. She particularly enjoyed the variety of recipes that kept her diet interesting. Emily's success was also attributed to her commitment to weekly meal planning and incorporating family-friendly recipes from the cookbook.

Case Study 3: Jessica's Triumph Over Health Issues

Jessica, a 50-year-old woman with a history of hormonal imbalances and slow metabolism, found relief with the Metabolic Confusion Diet. Within four months, she lost 20 pounds and noticed significant improvements in her hormonal health. Jessica's story is a testament to how the diet can help address underlying health issues that often hinder weight loss. By carefully monitoring her macronutrient intake and following the structured meal plans, Jessica achieved her health and weight goals.

TIPS FROM SUCCESSFUL DIETERS

- **Staying Consistent**

Consistency is key to success with the Metabolic Confusion Diet. Successful dieters like Sarah, Emily, and Jessica emphasize the importance of sticking to the meal plans and not skipping meals. They recommend setting reminders and keeping a food journal to track progress.

- **Embracing Variety**

Variety in meals prevents boredom and keeps motivation high. Emily advises experimenting with different recipes and not being afraid to try new ingredients. The cookbook's extensive range of recipes ensures there's something for everyone.

- **Planning Ahead**

Meal prepping and planning are crucial. Jessica suggests dedicating a day each week to prepare meals in advance. This not only saves time but also helps in making healthier choices.

- **Staying Hydrated**

Drinking plenty of water is essential for maintaining metabolism. Sarah found that staying hydrated helped her feel full and reduced cravings. Incorporating hydrating foods like fruits and vegetables also aids in staying on track.

<h1 style="text-align:center">MOTIVATIONAL STORIES</h1>

- **Overcoming Setbacks**

Every journey has its ups and downs. Emily faced setbacks during holidays and social events but learned to navigate them by making healthier choices and not being too hard on herself. She found that getting back on track quickly was more important than striving for perfection.

- **Celebrating Small Wins**

Celebrating small milestones keeps motivation high. Jessica celebrated every five-pound loss with non-food rewards like a new book or a spa day. Recognizing and rewarding progress helps maintain a positive mindset.

- **Building a Support System**

Having a support system is invaluable. Sarah joined online communities and forums where she shared her progress and challenges. The encouragement and advice from others on the same journey provided her with the motivation to continue.

The success stories of Sarah, Emily, and Jessica are just a few examples of how the Metabolic Confusion Diet can transform lives. Their journeys highlight the importance of consistency, variety, planning, hydration, and support.

By learning from these real-life transformations and incorporating the tips from successful dieters, readers can find inspiration and practical strategies to achieve their own health and weight loss goals.

28-DAY MEAL PLAN

WEEK 1

	BREAKFAST	LUNCH	DINNER
DAY 1	Avocado and Smoked Salmon Toast	Chicken Caesar Salad	Chicken Alfredo with Zoodles
DAY 2	Greek Yogurt Parfait	Turkey Lettuce Wraps	Shrimp and Veggie Stir-Fry
DAY 3	Quinoa Breakfast Bowl	Tuna and White Bean Salad	Turkey and Quinoa Stuffed Peppers
DAY 4	Peanut Butter Banana Smoothie	Vegetable and Hummus Wrap	Baked Salmon with Quinoa and Asparagus
DAY 5	Oatmeal with Nuts and Berries	Chickpea and Avocado Sandwich	Beef and Broccoli
DAY 6	Egg and Veggie Scramble	Lentil and Vegetable Stew	Stuffed Bell Peppers
DAY 7	Sweet Potato Hash	Quinoa and Black Bean Salad	Chicken and Pesto Pasta

WEEK 2

	BREAKFAST	LUNCH	DINNER
DAY 1	Green Smoothie	Zucchini Noodles with Pesto	Grilled Portobello Mushrooms
DAY 2	Chia Seed Pudding	Cabbage and Chicken Soup	Zoodle Pad Thai
DAY 3	Veggie Egg Muffins	Spinach and Feta Stuffed Mushrooms	Chicken Fajita Bowl
DAY 4	Protein-Packed Smoothie Bowl	Broccoli and Tofu Stir-Fry	Eggplant Parmesan
DAY 5	Cucumber and Tomato Salad	Cauliflower Fried Rice	Beef and Broccoli
DAY 6	Tofu Scramble	Greek Salad with Grilled Chicken	Salmon and Avocado Sushi Bowl
DAY 7	Sweet Potato Hash	Vegetable and Lentil Soup	Chicken and Veggie Kebabs

Repeat Week 1 and Week 2 to complete the 28-Day Meal Plan.
 Each week has a mix of lean proteins, complex carbohydrates, healthy fats, and fiber-rich foods to ensure optimal digestive health.

AVOCADO AND SMOKED SALMON TOAST

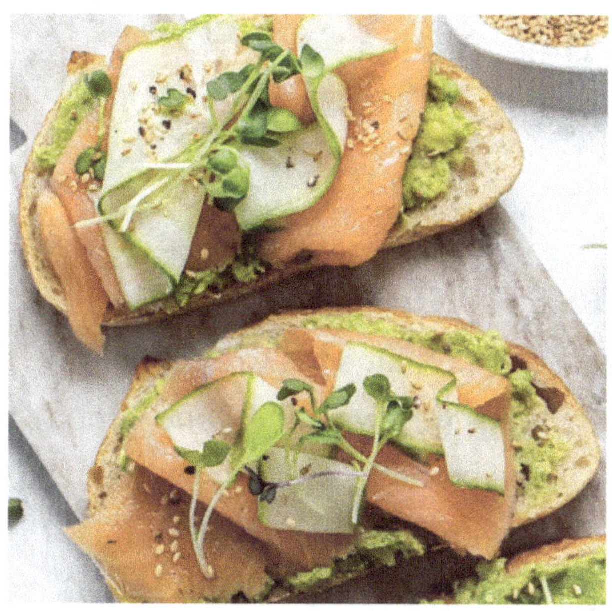

Prep Time: 15 Mins

Serving Size: 1

INGREDIENTS

- 2 slices of whole grain bread
- 1 ripe avocado
- 50g smoked salmon
- 1/4 cup of low-fat cream cheese
- 1 small tomato, sliced
- 1 tablespoon of lemon juice
- 1 tablespoon of chopped chives
- 1 teaspoon of capers
- Salt and pepper to taste
- Optional: red pepper flakes for added flavor
- Fresh lemon wedges for serving

INSTRUCTIONS

- Toast bread slices until crispy.
- Mash avocado with lemon juice, salt, and pepper.
- Mix cream cheese and chives.
- Spread mashed avocado on one slice of bread.
- Top with smoked salmon and capers.
- Spread cream cheese mixture on the other slice of bread.
- Top with tomato slices and red pepper flakes.
- Season with salt and pepper.
- Serve open-faced with lemon wedges.

NUTRITIONAL FACTS

- Calories: 400 kcal per serving
- Protein: 20g
- Carbohydrates: 35g
- Fat: 20g
- Fiber: 10g

GREEK YOGURT PARFAIT

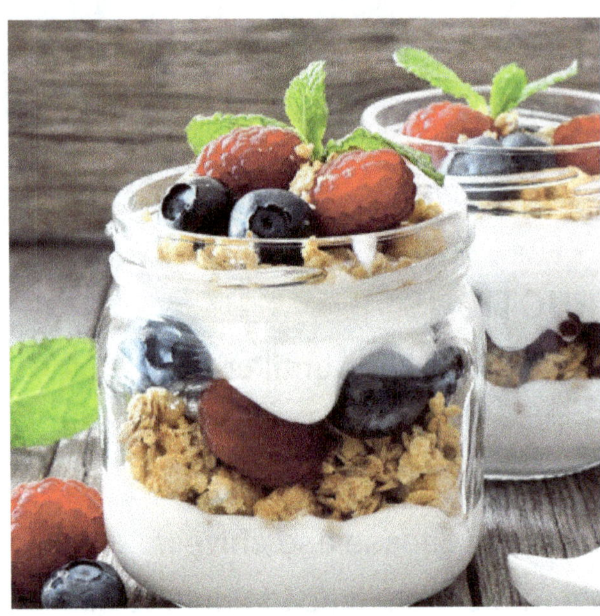

Prep Time: 5 Mins

Serving Size: 1

INGREDIENTS

- 1 cup plain full-fat Greek yogurt
- 1/4 cup mixed berries (blueberries, raspberries, strawberries)
- 1 tablespoon slivered almonds
- 1 teaspoon chia seeds
- 1 tablespoon honey or a low-calorie sweetener
- A pinch of lemon zest (optional)

INSTRUCTIONS

- In a bowl, combine the Greek yogurt with honey (or sweetener) and lemon zest until smooth.
- In a serving glass, place half of the yogurt mixture at the bottom.
- Add a layer of mixed berries on top of the yogurt.
- Sprinkle half of the almonds and chia seeds over the berries.
- Repeat the layers with the remaining yogurt, berries, almonds, and chia seeds.
- Garnish with a few berries and a touch of lemon zest for extra flavor.

NUTRITIONAL FACTS

- Calories: 280 kcal
- Protein: 22g
- Fats: 15g
- Carbohydrates: 18g

BERRY BLAST QUINOA BREAKFAST BOWL

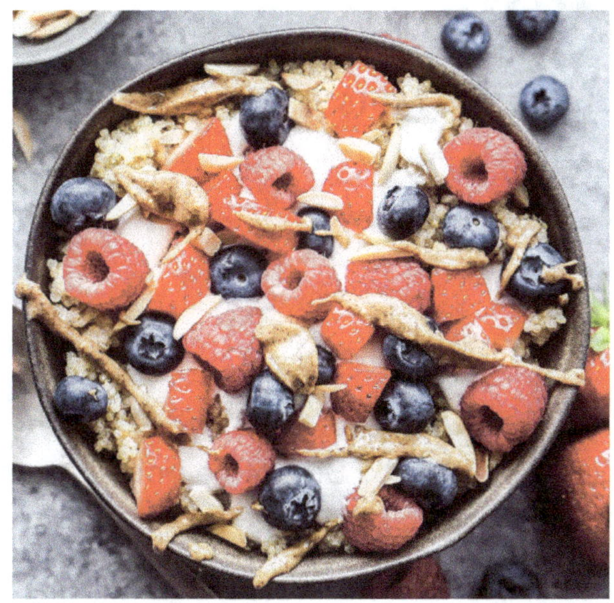

Cook Time: 25 Mins

Serving Size: 1

INGREDIENTS

- 1/2 cup quinoa, rinsed
- 1 cup water or almond milk
- 1/2 cup mixed berries (strawberries, blueberries, raspberries)
- 1 tablespoon honey or maple syrup
- 1 tablespoon almond butter
- 1 tablespoon chia seeds
- 1 tablespoon sliced almonds

INSTRUCTIONS

- In a small saucepan, bring water or almond milk to a boil.
- Add rinsed quinoa to the boiling liquid, reduce heat to low, cover, and simmer for 15-20 minutes or until quinoa is cooked and liquid is absorbed.
- Once quinoa is cooked, transfer it to a bowl.
- Top with mixed berries, almond butter, honey or maple syrup, chia seeds, and sliced almonds.
- Stir well to combine all ingredients.
- Enjoy your Berry Blast Quinoa Breakfast Bowl!

NUTRITIONAL FACTS

- Calories: 380 kcal
- Protein: 11g
- Carbohydrates: 58g
- Fat: 12g
- Fiber: 9g

TROPICAL PARADISE QUINOA BREAKFAST BOWL

Prep Time: 20 Mins

Serving Size: 1

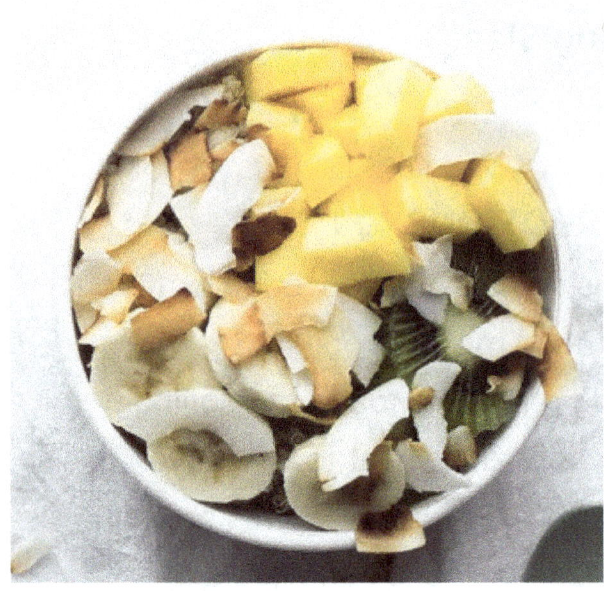

INGREDIENTS

- 1/2 cup quinoa, rinsed
- 1 cup coconut milk
- 1/2 banana, sliced
- 1/4 cup diced pineapple
- 1 tablespoon shredded coconut
- 1 tablespoon chopped macadamia nuts
- 1 teaspoon honey or agave syrup
- Pinch of cinnamon

INSTRUCTIONS

- In a small saucepan, combine quinoa and coconut milk. Bring to a boil.
- Reduce heat to low, cover, and simmer for 15-20 minutes, or until quinoa is cooked and liquid is absorbed.
- Once quinoa is cooked, transfer it to a bowl.
- Top with sliced banana, diced pineapple, shredded coconut, chopped macadamia nuts, honey or agave syrup, and a pinch of cinnamon.
- Stir well to combine.
- Enjoy your Tropical Paradise Quinoa Breakfast Bowl!

NUTRITIONAL FACTS

- Calories: 430 kcal
- Protein: 8g
- Carbohydrates: 51g
- Fat: 22g
- Fiber: 7g

PEANUT BUTTER BANANA SMOOTHIE

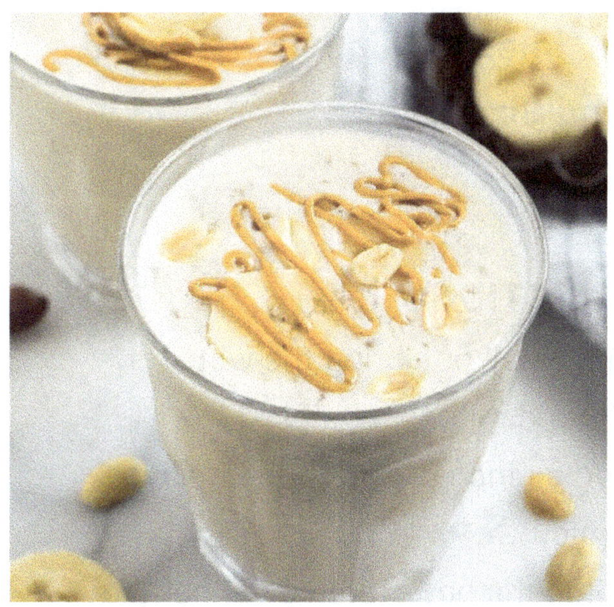

Prep Time: 5

Serving Size: 1

INGREDIENTS

- 1 medium ripe banana (approx. 100g)
- 2 tablespoons natural peanut butter (approx. 32g)
- 1 cup unsweetened almond milk (approx. 240ml)
- 1 scoop vanilla protein powder (approx. 30g)
- 1 tablespoon chia seeds (approx. 12g)
- 1 teaspoon honey (optional, approx. 7g)
- 1/2 teaspoon cinnamon
- 1/2 cup ice cube

INSTRUCTIONS

- Prepare Ingredients: Peel the banana and break it into chunks for easier blending.
- Blend: Add the banana, peanut butter, almond milk, protein powder, chia seeds, honey (if using), cinnamon, and ice cubes into a blender.
- Blend Until Smooth: Blend on high until the mixture is smooth and creamy.
- Serve: Pour the smoothie into a glass and serve immediately.

NUTRITIONAL FACTS

- Calories: 450
- Protein: 28g
- Fat: 20g
- Saturated Fat: 3g
- Carbohydrates: 47g
- Fiber: 8g
- Sugar: 22g

OATMEAL WITH NUTS AND BERRIES

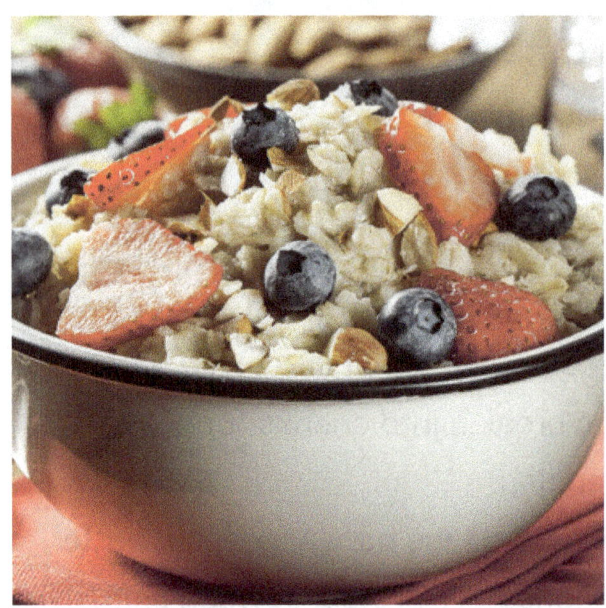

Cook Time: 10 Mins

Serving Size: 1

INGREDIENTS

- 1/2 cup old-fashioned oats
- 1 cup water or unsweetened almond milk
- 1/4 cup mixed berries (blueberries, strawberries, raspberries)
- 1 tablespoon chopped almonds
- 1 tablespoon chopped walnuts
- 1 teaspoon chia seeds
- 1 teaspoon honey or maple syrup (optional)
- 1/4 teaspoon ground cinnamon
- A pinch of salt

NUTRITIONAL FACTS

- Calories: 320kcal | Protein: 8g
- Carbohydrates: 44g | Fiber: 8g
- Sugars: 12g | Fat: 13g

INSTRUCTIONS

- In a small pot, bring the water or almond milk to a boil.
- Add a pinch of salt to the boiling liquid.
- Stir in the oats, reduce the heat to medium, and cook for about 5-7 minutes, stirring occasionally, until the oats have absorbed most of the liquid and reached your desired consistency.
- Stir in the ground cinnamon and let the oatmeal simmer for another minute.
- Transfer the cooked oatmeal to a bowl.
- Top with mixed berries, chopped almonds, chopped walnuts, and chia seeds.
- Drizzle with honey or maple syrup if desired for added sweetness.
- Enjoy your nutrient-packed oatmeal while it's warm.

TURKEY AND CHEESE OMELETTE

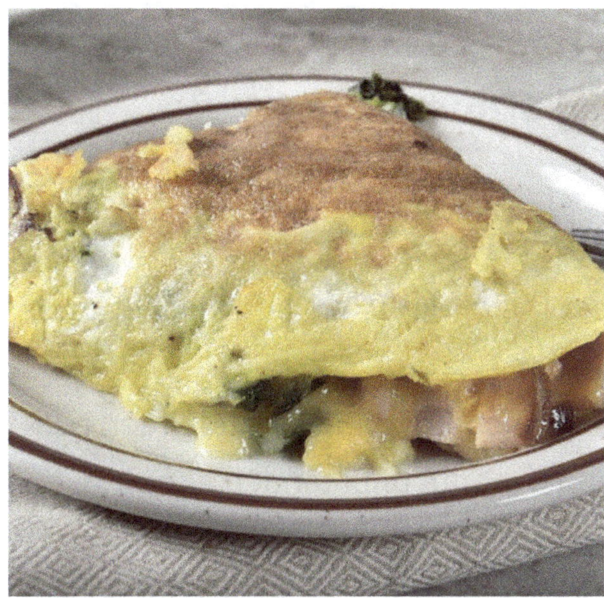

Cook Time: 10 Mins

Serving Size: 1

INGREDIENTS

- 3 large eggs
- 2 ounces of cooked turkey breast, shredded or chopped
- 1/4 cup shredded low-fat cheese (e.g., cheddar or mozzarella)
- 1/4 cup diced bell peppers
- 1/4 cup chopped spinach
- 1 small tomato, diced
- 1 tablespoon olive oil or cooking spray
- Salt and pepper to taste
- Optional: chopped herbs (e.g., parsley, chives) for garnish

INSTRUCTIONS

- Beat eggs with salt and pepper.
- Chop and dice the vegetables and turkey.
- Heat olive oil in a skillet over medium heat.
- Sauté bell peppers and spinach for 2-3 minutes.
- Pour in beaten eggs, cook until edges set.
- Add turkey and cheese on one half.
- Fold the omelette and cook until cheese melts.
- Slide omelette onto a plate.
- Garnish with diced tomatoes and herbs.
- Serve immediately.

NUTRITIONAL FACTS

- Calories: 350
- Protein: 28g
- Fat: 23g
- Carbohydrates: 5g
- Fiber: 1.5g
- Sugars: 3g

LOW-CALORIE TOFU SCRAMBLE

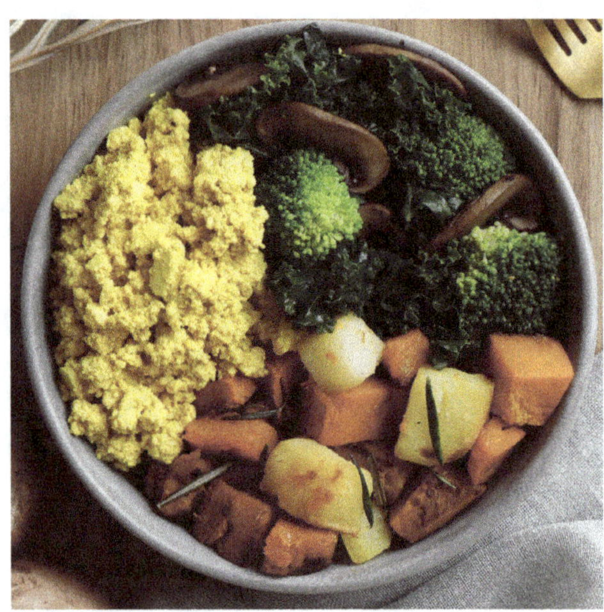

Cook Time: 20 Mins

Serving Size: 2

INGREDIENTS

- 1 block (14 oz) firm tofu, drained and crumbled
- 1 teaspoon olive oil
- 1 small onion, finely chopped
- 1 green bell pepper, diced
- 1/2 cup cherry tomatoes, halved
- 1 cup kale, chopped
- 1/4 cup nutritional yeast
- 1 teaspoon turmeric
- 1/2 teaspoon garlic powder
- Salt and pepper to taste
- 1 tablespoon lemon juice
- 2 tablespoons chopped fresh cilantro (optional)

INSTRUCTIONS

- Heat the olive oil in a large skillet over medium heat.
- Add the chopped onion and green bell pepper, sauté until tender, about 5 minutes.
- Crumble the tofu into the skillet and stir to combine.
- Add turmeric, garlic powder, salt, and pepper. Stir well to mix the spices evenly.
- Cook for 5-7 minutes, stirring occasionally, until the tofu is heated through.
- Add cherry tomatoes and kale, cook for another 2 minutes until kale is wilted.
- Remove from heat and stir in the nutritional yeast and lemon juice.
- Top with fresh cilantro if using.
- Serve hot.

NUTRITIONAL FACTS

- Calories: 210kcal | Protein: 20g
- Carbohydrates: 12g | Fat: 11g
- Fiber: 6g

GRILLED CHICKEN AND AVOCADO SALAD

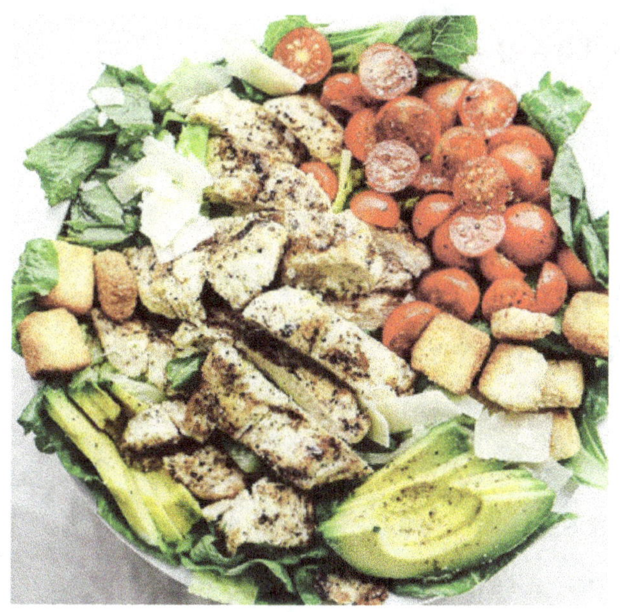

Cook Time: 15 Mins

Serving Size: 2

INGREDIENTS

- 2 boneless, skinless chicken breasts (about 6 ounces each)
- 1 tablespoon olive oil
- 1 teaspoon garlic powder
- 1 teaspoon paprika
- Salt and pepper to taste
- 1 avocado, diced
- 4 cups mixed salad greens (e.g., spinach, arugula, romaine)
- 1 cup cherry tomatoes, halved
- 1 small cucumber, sliced
- 1/4 red onion, thinly sliced
- 1/4 cup crumbled feta cheese
- 2 tablespoons balsamic vinaigrette

INSTRUCTIONS

- In a small bowl, mix olive oil, garlic powder, paprika, salt, and pepper.
- Rub the chicken breasts with the spice mixture and let them marinate for about 10 minutes.
- Preheat the grill to medium-high heat.
- Grill the chicken breasts for 6-7 minutes on each side, or until the internal temperature reaches 165°F (75°C).
- Once cooked, remove the chicken from the grill and let it rest for 5 minutes before slicing.
- In a large salad bowl, combine mixed salad greens, cherry tomatoes, cucumber, red onion, and crumbled feta cheese.
- Add the diced avocado.
- Slice the grilled chicken breasts and place them on top of the salad.
- Drizzle with balsamic vinaigrette.
- Toss the salad gently to combine the ingredients and serve immediately.

TURKEY AND QUINOA STUFFED PEPPERS

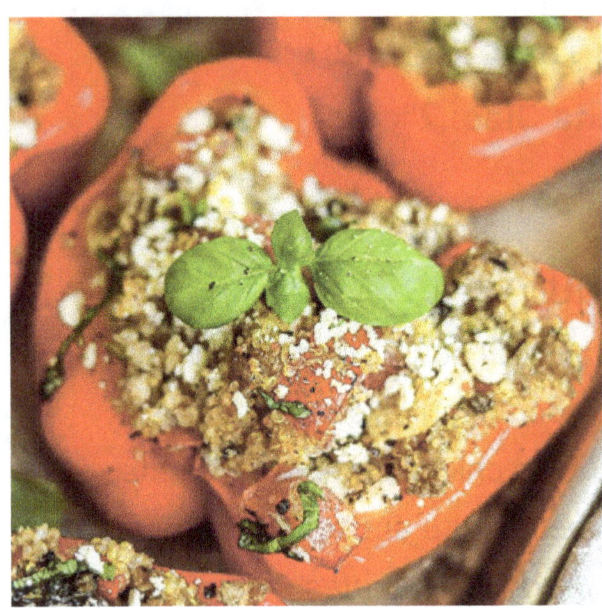

Prep Time: 45 Mins

Serving Size: 4

INGREDIENTS

- 4 large bell peppers (any color)
- 1 lb (450g) lean ground turkey
- 1 cup cooked quinoa
- 1 small onion, finely chopped
- 2 cloves garlic, minced
- 1 can (14.5 oz) diced tomatoes, drained
- 1 cup spinach, chopped
- 1 tsp cumin
- 1 tsp smoked paprika
- 1 tsp dried oregano
- Salt and pepper to taste
- 1 cup shredded low-fat mozzarella cheese (optional)
- 1 tbsp olive oil
- Fresh parsley or cilantro for garnish (optional)

INSTRUCTIONS

- Preheat oven to 375°F (190°C).
- Cut tops off bell peppers, remove seeds, and coat with olive oil. Place cut side up in a baking dish.
- If not already cooked, prepare quinoa according to package instructions.
- Heat olive oil in a skillet over medium heat. Sauté onion and garlic until soft.
- Add ground turkey and cook until browned.
- Stir in tomatoes, spinach, spices, salt, and pepper. Cook until spinach is wilted. Mix in cooked quinoa.
- Fill each bell pepper with the turkey-quinoa mixture.
- Cover with foil and bake for 30 minutes. Remove foil, top with cheese (if using), and bake for an additional 10 minutes.
- Let cool slightly, garnish with parsley or cilantro, and serve warm.

BEEF AND BROCCOLI STIR-FRY

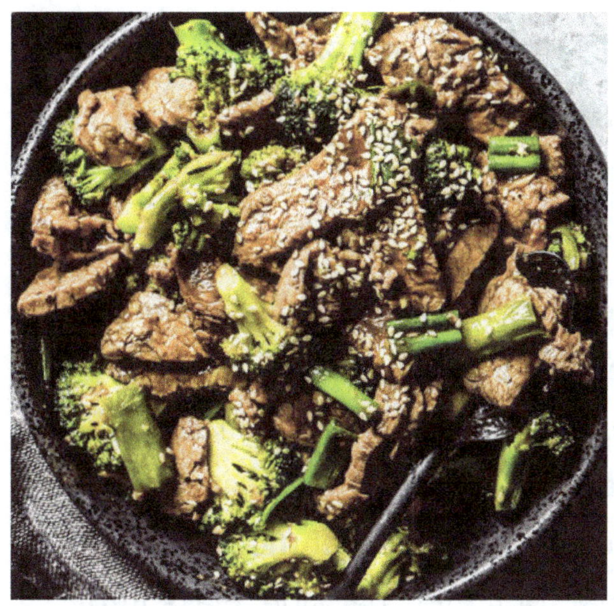

Cook Time: 20 Mins

Serving Size: 4

INGREDIENTS

- 1 lb beef sirloin, thinly sliced
- 3 cups broccoli florets
- 2 Tbsp olive oil
- 1 Tbsp minced garlic
- 1/2 cup low-sodium beef broth
- 2 Tbsp low-sodium soy sauce
- 1 Tbsp oyster sauce
- 1 tsp cornstarch
- 1 tsp sesame oil
- Salt and pepper to taste

NUTRITIONAL FACTS

- Calories: 260kcal | Protein: 24g
- Carbohydrates: 10g | Fiber: 3g
- Sugars: 2g
- Fat: 13g

INSTRUCTIONS

- In a small bowl, combine the beef broth, soy sauce, oyster sauce, cornstarch, and sesame oil. Whisk until well blended and set aside.
- Heat the olive oil in a large skillet over medium-high heat. Add the minced garlic and sauté for about 30 seconds until fragrant.
- Add the thinly sliced beef to the skillet and stir-fry until browned, then remove from the skillet and set aside.
- In the same skillet, add the broccoli florets and stir-fry until they are bright green and tender-crisp.
- Return the cooked beef to the skillet with the broccoli.
- Pour the sauce mixture over the beef and broccoli, stirring well to coat everything evenly. Cook for an additional 2-3 minutes until the sauce thickens.
- Season with salt and pepper to taste before serving.

SALMON AND AVOCADO SUSHI BOWL

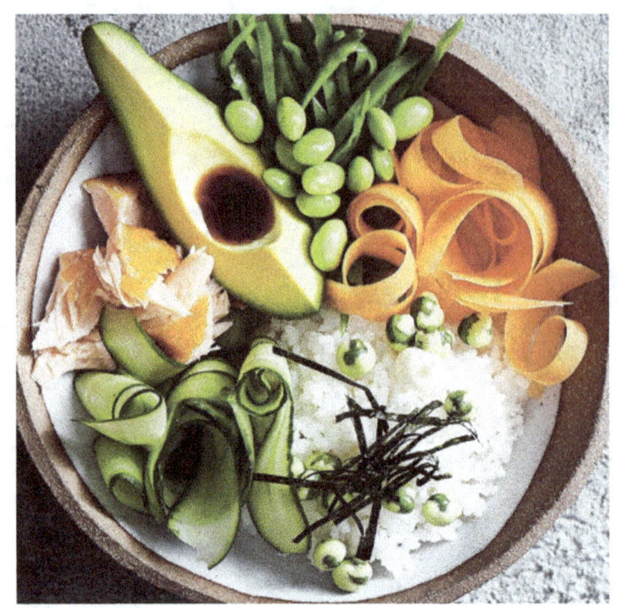

Cook Time: 30 Mins

Serving Size: 2

INSTRUCTIONS

- Cook cauliflower rice in a skillet until tender (5 mins). Cook quinoa according to package instructions.
- Season salmon with salt and pepper. Cook in a skillet over medium-high heat for 4 mins per side. Flake into pieces.
- Julienne cucumber and carrot. Slice avocado.
- Divide quinoa and cauliflower rice between two bowls. Top with salmon, avocado, cucumber, carrot, edamame, and pickled ginger. Drizzle with soy sauce, rice vinegar, and sesame oil. Garnish with sesame seeds, green onions, and nori strips.

INGREDIENTS

- 200g fresh salmon fillet
- 1 medium avocado
- 1/2 cup cooked quinoa
- 1/2 cup cauliflower rice
- 1 small cucumber
- 1 small carrot
- 1/2 cup edamame (shelled)
- 1 tablespoon soy sauce (low sodium)
- 1 tablespoon rice vinegar
- 1 teaspoon sesame oil
- 1 teaspoon sesame seeds
- 1 sheet nori (seaweed), cut into thin strips
- 1 tablespoon pickled ginger
- 1 tablespoon green onions, chopped
- Salt and pepper to taste

NUTRITIONAL FACTS

- Calories: 385kcal
- Protein: 29g
- Carbohydrates: 25g
- Fat: 19g
- Fiber: 7.5g

MEDITERRANEAN TUNA AND WHITE BEAN SALAD

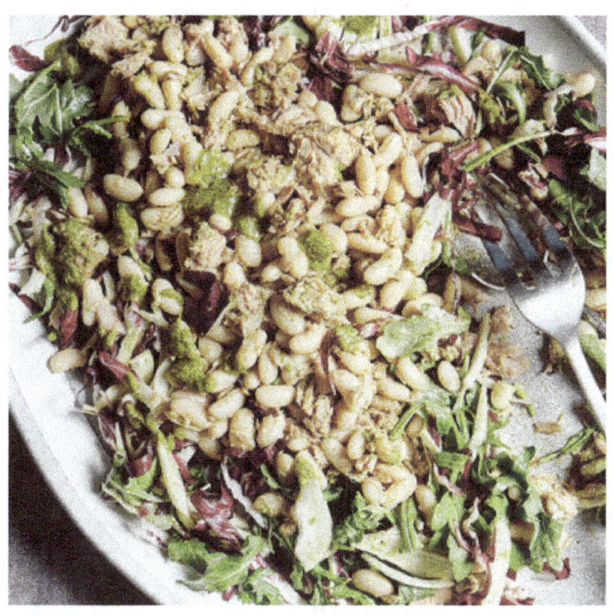

INGREDIENTS

- 1 can (5 oz) tuna packed in water, drained
- 1 can (15 oz) white beans (cannellini or navy beans), drained and rinsed
- 1 cup cherry tomatoes, halved
- 1/2 cup red onion, finely chopped
- 1/4 cup kalamata olives, pitted and sliced
- 1/4 cup fresh parsley, chopped
- 2 cups mixed greens (arugula, spinach, or your choice)
- 2 tbsp extra virgin olive oil
- 1 tbsp red wine vinegar
- 1 tsp lemon zest
- Salt and pepper to taste

Cook Time: 15 Mins

Serving Size: 2

INSTRUCTIONS

- In a large bowl, combine the drained tuna, white beans, cherry tomatoes, red onion, olives, and parsley.
- In a small bowl, whisk together the olive oil, red wine vinegar, lemon zest, salt, and pepper.
- Pour the dressing over the salad and toss gently to combine.
- Serve the salad over a bed of mixed greens.

NUTRITIONAL FACTS

- Calories: 350kcal
- Protein: 25g
- Carbohydrates: 30g
- Fat: 15g
- Fiber: 8g

AVOCADO TUNA AND WHITE BEAN SALAD

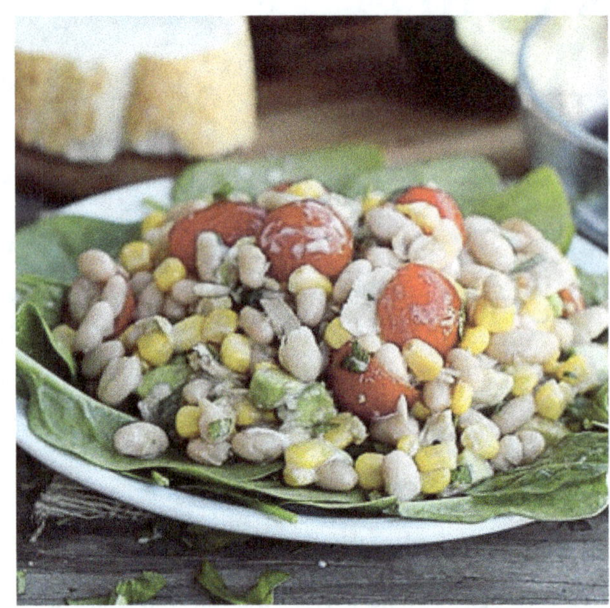

Cook Time: 15 Mins

Serving Size: 2

INSTRUCTIONS

- In a large bowl, combine the drained tuna, white beans, avocado, cherry tomatoes, red onion, and cilantro.
- In a small bowl, whisk together the lime juice, olive oil, salt, and pepper.
- Pour the dressing over the salad and toss gently to combine.
- Serve immediately.

INGREDIENTS

- 1 can (5 oz) tuna packed in water, drained
- 1 can (15 oz) white beans (cannellini or great northern), drained and rinsed
- 1 avocado, diced
- 1/2 cup cherry tomatoes, halved
- 1/4 cup red onion, finely chopped
- 1/4 cup cilantro, chopped
- 1 lime, juiced
- 2 tbsp extra virgin olive oil
- Salt and pepper to taste

NUTRITIONAL FACTS

- Calories: 370
- Protein: 22g
- Carbohydrates: 30g
- Fat: 20g
- Fiber: 10g

TURKEY LETTUCE WRAPS

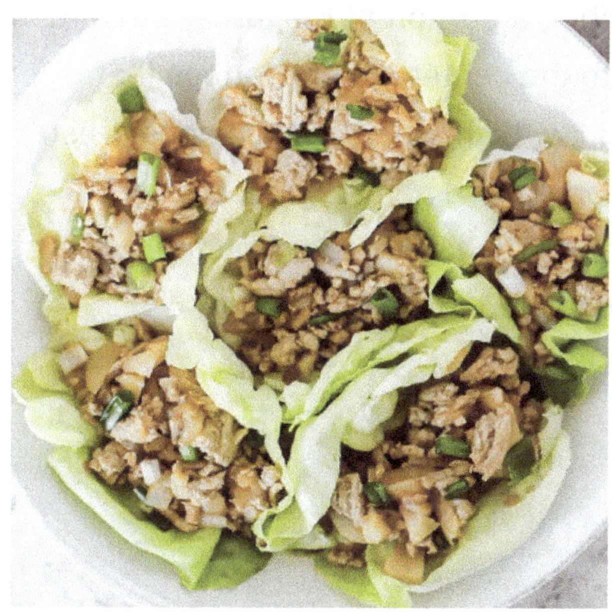

INGREDIENTS

- 1 lb (450g) ground turkey
- 1 tablespoon olive oil
- 1 small onion, finely chopped
- 2 cloves garlic, minced
- 1 red bell pepper, finely chopped
- 1 cup shredded carrots
- 1/4 cup hoisin sauce
- 2 tablespoons soy sauce (low sodium)
- 1 tablespoon rice vinegar
- 1 teaspoon ginger, grated
- 1 teaspoon sriracha sauce (optional for spice)
- 8 large lettuce leaves (Boston Bibb or Butter Lettuce works best)
- 2 green onions, chopped

Cook Time: 24 Mins

Serving Size: 4

INSTRUCTIONS

- Wash and dry the lettuce leaves, set aside.
- Finely chop the onion, red bell pepper, and shred the carrots.
- Heat the olive oil in a large skillet over medium-high heat.
- Add the chopped onion and cook until it becomes translucent, about 3-4 minutes.
- Add the garlic and cook for another minute until fragrant.
- Add the ground turkey to the skillet, breaking it up with a spoon, and cook until it's no longer pink, about 5-7 minutes.
- Stir in the red bell pepper and shredded carrots, cooking until they soften, about 3-4 minutes.
- In a small bowl, mix together the hoisin sauce, soy sauce, rice vinegar, grated ginger, and sriracha sauce (if using). Pour the sauce into the skillet and stir to combine, cooking for another 2-3 minutes to let the flavors meld.

INGREDIENTS

- 1/4 cup fresh cilantro, chopped
- 1/4 cup peanuts, chopped (optional)
- Lime wedges for serving

NUTRITIONAL FACTS

- Calories: 210kcal
- Protein: 20g
- Carbohydrates: 12g
- Fiber: 3g
- Sugars: 6g
- Fat: 10g

INSTRUCTIONS

- Spoon a portion of the turkey mixture into the center of each lettuce leaf.
- Top with chopped green onions, fresh cilantro, and peanuts if desired.
- Serve with lime wedges on the side for an added zesty flavor.

SPICY VEGGIE AND HUMMUS WRAP

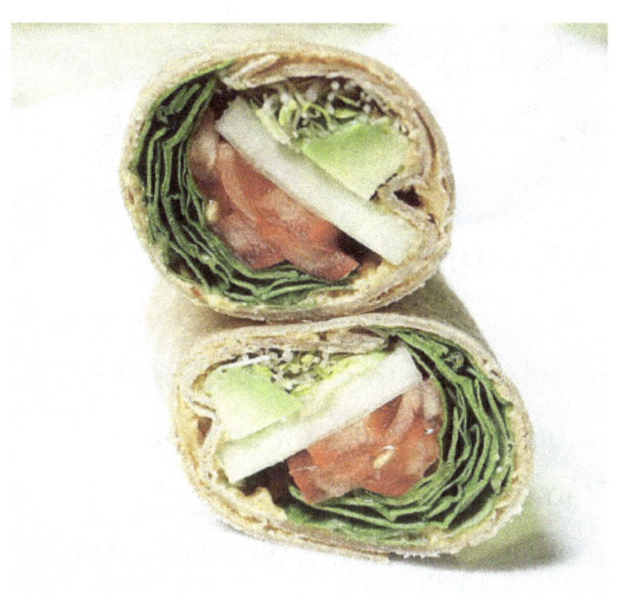

Cook Time: 15 Mins

Serving Size: 1

INSTRUCTIONS

- Spread the spicy hummus evenly over the tortilla.
- Layer the shredded purple cabbage, julienned carrots, and sliced bell peppers on top of the hummus.
- Add the baby kale, jalapeños, and avocado slices.
- Drizzle with lime juice and season with salt and pepper.
- Roll the tortilla tightly, tucking in the sides as you go.
- Slice in half and serve.

INGREDIENTS

- 1 whole wheat tortilla or wrap
- 3 tablespoons spicy hummus
- 1/4 cup shredded purple cabbage
- 1/4 cup julienned carrots
- 1/4 cup sliced bell peppers (red or yellow)
- 1/4 cup baby kale
- 1 tablespoon sliced jalapeños (optional)
- 1/4 avocado, sliced
- 1 teaspoon lime juice
- Salt and pepper to taste

NUTRITIONAL FACTS

- Calories: 310kcal
- Protein: 7g
- Carbohydrates: 39g
- Fiber: 11g
- Fat: 14g

CHICKPEA AND AVOCADO SALAD SANDWICH

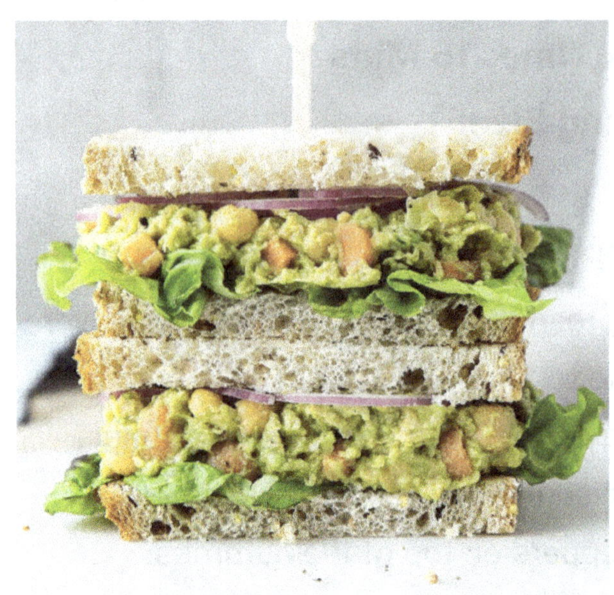

Cook Time: 20

Serving Size: 1

INSTRUCTIONS

- In a medium bowl, mash the avocado and chickpeas together until well combined but still a bit chunky.
- Stir in the Greek yogurt, Dijon mustard, lemon juice, diced celery, and diced red bell pepper.
- Season with salt and pepper to taste.
- Toast the whole grain bread slices if desired.
- Spread the avocado and chickpea salad evenly over one slice of bread.
- Top with lettuce leaves if using.
- Place the second slice of bread on top to complete the sandwich.
- Cut in half and serve.

INGREDIENTS

- 2 slices whole grain bread
- 1/2 ripe avocado
- 1/2 cup canned chickpeas, drained and rinsed
- 1 tablespoon plain Greek yogurt
- 1 teaspoon Dijon mustard
- 1 teaspoon lemon juice
- 1/4 cup diced celery
- 1/4 cup diced red bell pepper
- Salt and pepper to taste
- Lettuce leaves (optional)

NUTRITIONAL FACTS

- Calories: 360kcal
- Protein: 11g
- Carbohydrates: 42g
- Dietary Fiber: 12g
- Sugars: 5g
- Fat: 18g

ZUCCHINI NOODLES WITH PESTO

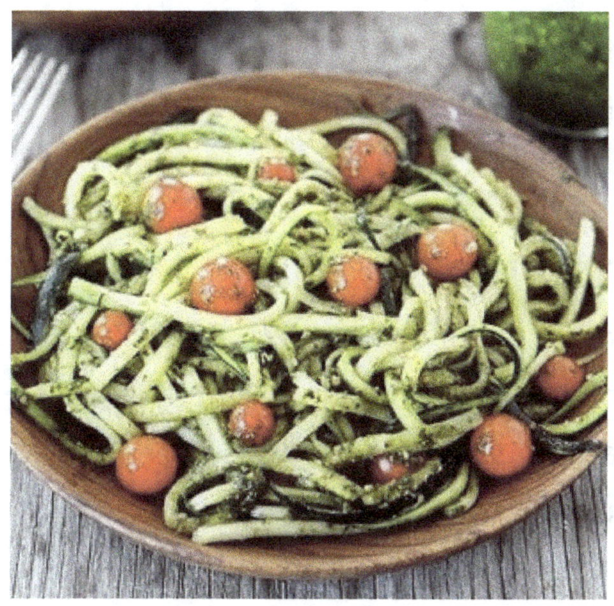

INGREDIENTS

- 2 medium-sized zucchinis
- 1 cup fresh basil leaves
- 1/4 cup pine nuts
- 2 cloves garlic, minced
- 1/4 cup grated Parmesan cheese (optional, can be omitted for a dairy-free version)
- 1/4 cup extra virgin olive oil
- Salt and pepper to taste
- Optional toppings: cherry tomatoes, grilled chicken, or shrimp

NUTRITIONAL FACTS

- Calories: 320kcal | Fat: 30g
- Carbohydrates: 8g | Fiber: 3g
- Sugars: 4g | Protein: 8g

Cook Time: 20 Mins

Serving Size: 2

INSTRUCTIONS

- Using a spiralizer or a vegetable peeler, create zucchini noodles. Set aside.
- In a food processor, combine the basil leaves, pine nuts, garlic, and Parmesan cheese (if using). Pulse until finely chopped. While the food processor is running, slowly drizzle in the olive oil until the mixture is smooth. Season with salt and pepper to taste.
- In a large skillet, heat a drizzle of olive oil over medium heat. Add the zucchini noodles and sauté for 2-3 minutes until they are just tender but still have a slight crunch.
- Once the zucchini noodles are cooked, add the pesto to the skillet and toss until the noodles are evenly coated.
- Divide the zucchini noodles with pesto between two plates. Top with optional toppings such as cherry tomatoes, grilled chicken, or shrimp if desired.

BAKED SWEET POTATO FRIES

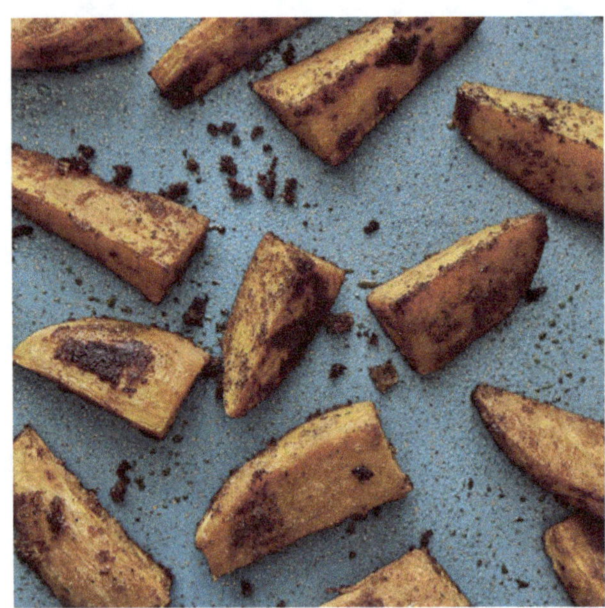

Cook Time: 30 Mins

Serving Size: 2

INGREDIENTS

- 2 medium sweet potatoes, washed and peeled
- 2 tablespoons olive oil
- 1 teaspoon paprika
- 1 teaspoon garlic powder
- 1/2 teaspoon cumin
- Salt and pepper to taste
- Optional: chopped parsley for garnish

NUTRITIONAL FACTS

- Calories: 200 kcal
- Total Fat: 7g
- Carbohydrates: 32g
- Fiber: 5g | Sugars: 6g
- Protein: 2g

INSTRUCTIONS

- Preheat your oven to 425°F (220°C) and line a baking sheet with parchment paper.
- Cut the sweet potatoes into thin strips, resembling fries.
- In a large bowl, toss the sweet potato strips with olive oil, paprika, garlic powder, cumin, salt, and pepper until evenly coated.
- Spread the sweet potato fries in a single layer on the prepared baking sheet, making sure they're not overcrowded.
- Bake in the preheated oven for 25-30 minutes, flipping halfway through, until the fries are crispy and golden brown.
- Once done, remove from the oven and sprinkle with chopped parsley if desired.
- Serve immediately and enjoy!

CHICKEN AND PESTO PASTA

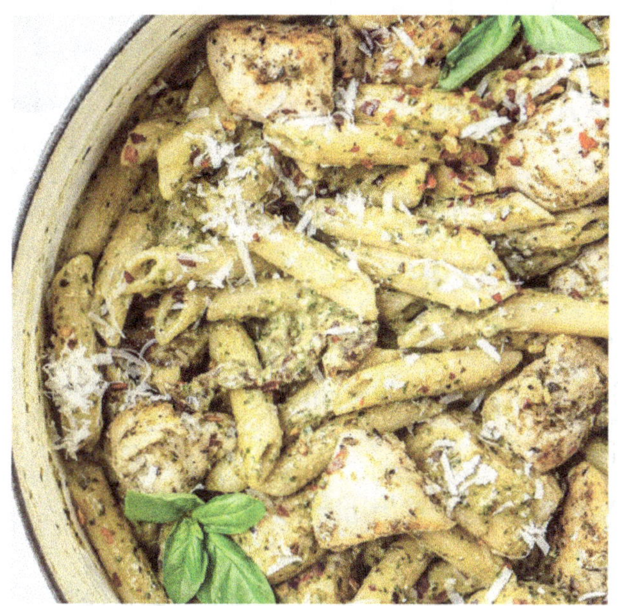

INGREDIENTS

- 8 oz whole wheat pasta
- 2 boneless, skinless chicken breasts, thinly sliced
- 2 tablespoons olive oil
- 2 cloves garlic, minced
- 1 cup cherry tomatoes, halved
- 2 cups spinach leaves
- ¼ cup basil pesto
- Salt and pepper to taste
- Grated Parmesan cheese for garnish (optional)

NUTRITIONAL FACTS

- Calories: 380kcal
- Protein: 25g
- Carbohydrates: 35g
- Fat: 16g
- Fiber: 6g

INSTRUCTIONS

- Cook the pasta according to package instructions until al dente. Drain and set aside.
- In a large skillet, heat 1 tablespoon of olive oil over medium-high heat. Add the sliced chicken breasts and cook until browned and cooked through, about 5-6 minutes per side. Remove the chicken from the skillet and set aside.
- In the same skillet, add the remaining tablespoon of olive oil. Add the minced garlic and cook for 1-2 minutes until fragrant.
- Add the cherry tomatoes to the skillet and cook for 2-3 minutes until they start to soften.
- Return the cooked chicken to the skillet. Add the spinach leaves and cooked pasta. Stir in the basil pesto until everything is well coated and heated through.
- Season with salt and pepper to taste.
- Serve hot, garnished with grated Parmesan cheese if desired.

SHRIMP AND VEGGIE STIR-FRY

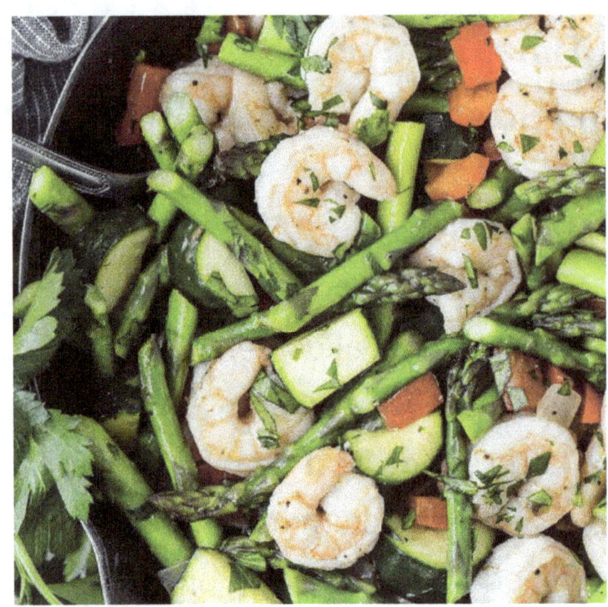

Cook Time: 20 Mins

Serving Size: 2

INGREDIENTS

- 1/2 pound large shrimp, peeled and deveined
- 2 cups mixed vegetables (broccoli florets, bell peppers, snap peas, carrots), sliced
- 2 cloves garlic, minced
- 1 tablespoon ginger, minced
- 2 tablespoons low-sodium soy sauce or tamari
- 1 tablespoon rice vinegar
- 1 tablespoon sesame oil
- 1 teaspoon honey or maple syrup
- 1 tablespoon olive oil or coconut oil
- Salt and pepper to taste
- Optional: Red pepper flakes for added spice
- Cooked quinoa or brown rice for serving (optional)

INSTRUCTIONS

- **Prepare Ingredients:** Peel shrimp, chop veggies, and mince garlic and ginger.
- **Make Sauce:** Whisk soy sauce, rice vinegar, sesame oil, and honey.
- **Cook Shrimp:** Sauté shrimp until pink, then set aside.
- **Sauté Aromatics and Veggies:** Sauté garlic, ginger, and veggies until tender.
- **Combine:** Add shrimp back to the skillet, pour sauce, and toss.
- **Serve:** Season, then serve alone or with quinoa/rice.

NUTRITIONAL FACTS

- Calories: 250 kcal
- Protein: 20g
- Carbohydrates: 15g
- Fat: 12g
- Fiber: 4g

TURKEY MEATBALLS

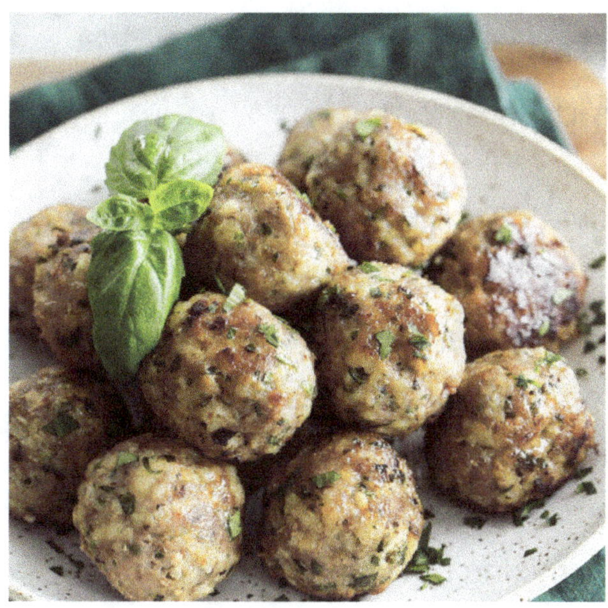

Cook Time: 30 Mins

Serving Size: 4

INGREDIENTS

- 1 lb lean ground turkey
- 1/4 cup almond flour
- 1/4 cup grated Parmesan cheese
- 1/4 cup chopped fresh parsley
- 1/4 cup finely chopped onion
- 2 cloves garlic, minced
- 1 teaspoon dried oregano
- 1 teaspoon dried basil
- 1/2 teaspoon salt
- 1/4 teaspoon black pepper
- 1 egg
- Cooking spray

NUTRITIONAL FACTS

- Calories: 250 kcal | Protein: 25g
- Carbohydrates: 5g | Fat: 14g
- Fiber: 1g

INSTRUCTIONS

- Preheat your oven to 180°C (350°F).
- In a large mixing bowl, combine the lean ground beef, chopped onion, minced garlic, rolled oats, grated zucchini, grated carrot, chopped parsley, eggs, and milk.
- Season the mixture with salt and pepper according to your taste preferences.
- Mix all the ingredients thoroughly until well combined.
- Lightly grease a muffin tin with cooking spray or olive oil.
- Spoon the meat mixture evenly into the muffin tin, filling each cup about 3/4 full.
- Place the muffin tin in the preheated oven and bake for 25-30 minutes, or until the meat muffins are cooked through and golden brown on top.
- Once cooked, remove the muffin tin from the oven and let the meaty muffins cool for a few minutes before serving.

BAKED COD WITH ROASTED VEGGIES

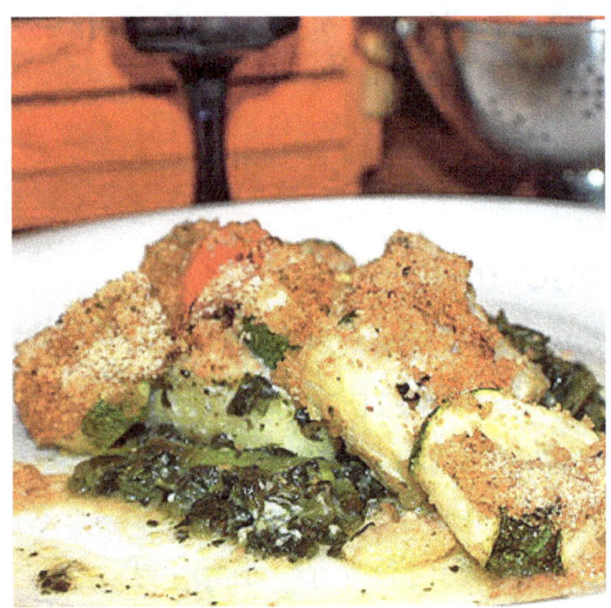

Prep Time: 35 Mins

Serving Size: 2

INGREDIENTS

- 2 cod fillets (about 6 oz each)
- 2 cups mixed vegetables (such as bell peppers, zucchini, cherry tomatoes, and red onion), chopped
- 2 tablespoons olive oil
- 2 cloves garlic, minced
- 1 teaspoon dried thyme
- 1 teaspoon dried rosemary
- Salt and pepper to taste
- Lemon wedges for serving

NUTRITIONAL FACTS

- Calories: 320 kcal
- Protein: 30g
- Carbohydrates: 14g
- Fat: 16g
- Fiber: 4g

INSTRUCTIONS

- Preheat your oven to 400°F (200°C).
- Prepare a baking sheet by lining it with parchment paper or lightly greasing it with olive oil.
- In a mixing bowl, toss the chopped vegetables with olive oil, minced garlic, dried thyme, dried rosemary, salt, and pepper until well coated.
- Spread the seasoned vegetables evenly on the prepared baking sheet.
- Place the cod fillets on top of the vegetables.
- Season the cod fillets with salt, pepper, and a drizzle of olive oil.
- Bake in the preheated oven for 20-25 minutes, or until the cod is cooked through and flakes easily with a fork.
- Once done, remove from the oven and let it rest for a few minutes.
- Serve the baked cod with roasted veggies hot, with lemon wedges on the side for squeezing over the fish.

HARD BOILED EGGS

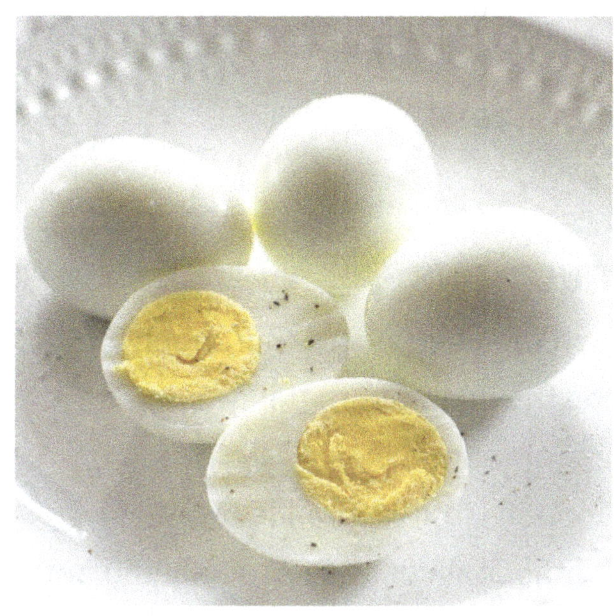

Cook Time: 12 Mins

Serving Size: 2

INSTRUCTIONS

- Prepare: Place eggs in a pot, cover with water.
- Boil: Bring to a rolling boil over high heat.
- Cook: Cover pot, remove from heat, let sit for 9-12 minutes.
- Cool: Transfer eggs to an ice bath for 5 minutes.
- Peel and Serve: Peel under running water.

INGREDIENTS

- 4 large eggs
- Water (enough to cover the eggs in the pot)
- Ice cubes (for the ice bath)

NUTRITIONAL FACTS

- Calories: 140kcal
- Protein: 12g
- Fat: 10g
- Saturated Fat: 3g
- Carbohydrates: 1g
- Fiber: 0g
- Sugars: 0g

CUCUMBER SLICES WITH TZATZIKI

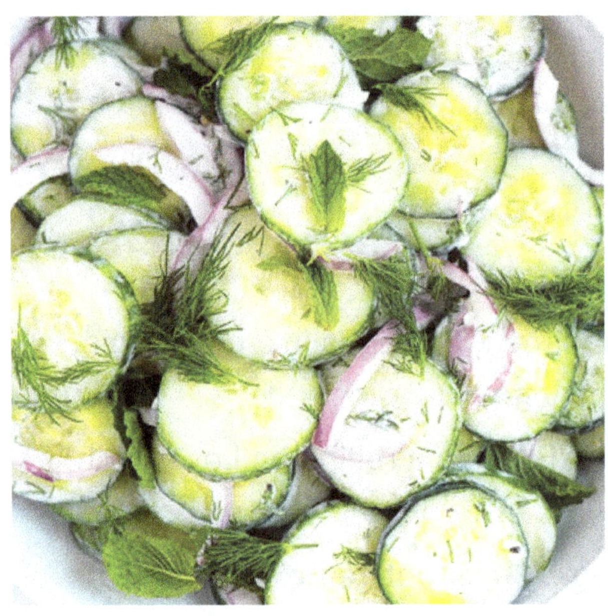

Cook Time: 30 Mins

Serving Size: 4

INGREDIENTS

For the Cucumber Slices:
- 2 large cucumbers, sliced thinly
- 1/4 teaspoon sea salt (optional)

For the Tzatziki:
- 1 cup Greek yogurt (full-fat or 2%)
- 1 medium cucumber, grated and excess water squeezed out
- 2 cloves garlic, minced
- 1 tablespoon fresh lemon juice
- 1 tablespoon extra virgin olive oil
- 1 tablespoon fresh dill, chopped (or 1 teaspoon dried dill)
- 1/2 teaspoon sea salt
- 1/4 teaspoon black pepper

INSTRUCTIONS

- Wash the cucumbers thoroughly.
- Slice the cucumbers thinly using a knife or mandoline.
- Optional: Lightly sprinkle the cucumber slices with sea salt and set aside for 10 minutes to draw out excess moisture. Pat dry with a paper towel.
- Grate the cucumber and squeeze out the excess water using a cheesecloth or paper towels.
- In a medium bowl, combine the Greek yogurt, grated cucumber, minced garlic, lemon juice, olive oil, dill, sea salt, and black pepper.
- Mix well until all ingredients are fully incorporated.
- Cover and refrigerate the tzatziki for at least 30 minutes to allow the flavors to meld together.
- Arrange the cucumber slices on a serving platter.
- Serve the cucumber slices with a side of tzatziki for dipping.

ZOODLE PAD THAI

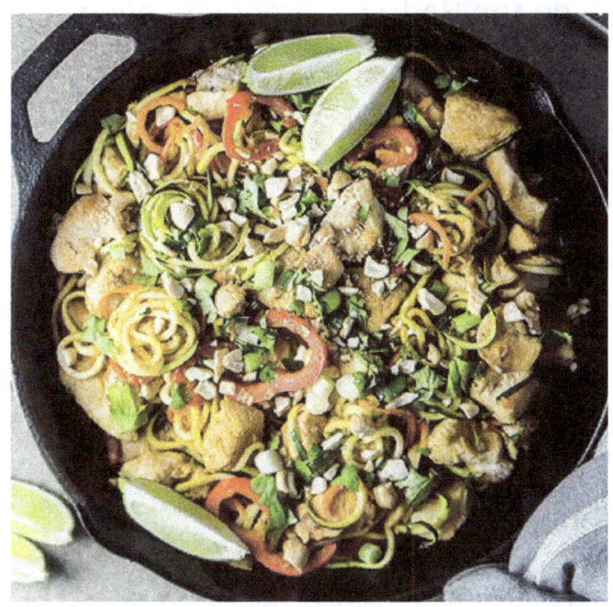

Cook Time: 20 Mins

Serving Size: 2

INGREDIENTS

- 2 medium zucchinis, spiralized into noodles
- 1 tablespoon coconut oil
- 1 small onion, thinly sliced
- 2 cloves garlic, minced
- 1 small carrot, julienned
- 1 small red bell pepper, thinly sliced
- 1 cup bean sprouts
- 2 eggs, beaten
- 2 tablespoons chopped peanuts (optional, for garnish)
- 2 green onions, sliced (optional, for garnish)
- Fresh cilantro leaves (optional, for garnish)
- Lime wedges (optional, for serving)

INSTRUCTIONS

- In a small bowl, whisk together all the sauce ingredients until well combined. Set aside.
- Heat coconut oil in a large skillet over medium heat. Add onion and garlic, sauté for 2-3 minutes until softened. Add carrot, bell pepper, and bean sprouts, and cook for another 2-3 minutes until vegetables are tender-crisp.
- Push the vegetables to one side of the skillet and add the beaten eggs to the other side. Scramble the eggs until cooked through, then mix with the vegetables.
- Add the zucchini noodles (zoodles) to the skillet along with the prepared sauce. Toss everything together until the zoodles are coated with the sauce and heated through, about 2-3 minutes.

INGREDIENTS

Sauce:

- 3 tablespoons low-sodium soy sauce
- 2 tablespoons lime juice
- 1 tablespoon honey or maple syrup
- 1 tablespoon rice vinegar
- 1 teaspoon Sriracha sauce (adjust to taste)
- 1 teaspoon grated ginger

NUTRITIONAL FACTS

- Calories: 250 kcal
- Protein: 10g
- Carbohydrates: 25g
- Fat: 12g
- Fiber: 5g
- Sugar: 10g

INSTRUCTIONS

- Divide the Pad Thai among serving plates. Garnish with chopped peanuts, green onions, cilantro leaves, and lime wedges if desired.

CAULIFLOWER FRIED RICE

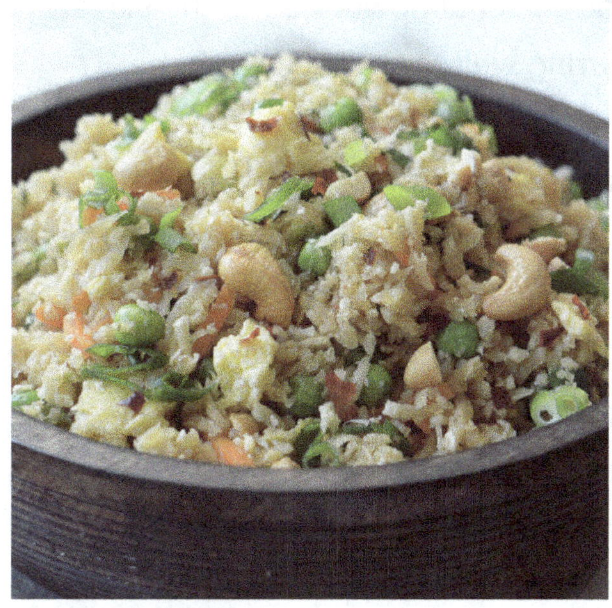

Cook Time: 20 Mins

Serving Size: 4

INGREDIENTS

- 1 medium head cauliflower, grated or riced
- 2 tablespoons olive oil
- 2 cloves garlic, minced
- 1 small onion, diced
- 1 cup mixed vegetables (such as peas, carrots, bell peppers)
- 2 eggs, lightly beaten
- 2 tablespoons low-sodium soy sauce (or tamari for gluten-free option)
- 1 teaspoon sesame oil
- Salt and pepper to taste
- Optional: cooked chicken, shrimp, or tofu for added protein
- Optional garnishes: chopped green onions, sesame seeds

INSTRUCTIONS

- Prepare the cauliflower by removing the stems and leaves. Cut into florets and either pulse in a food processor until it resembles rice or grate using a box grater. Set aside.
- Heat olive oil in a large skillet or wok over medium heat. Add minced garlic and diced onion, sauté until fragrant and onions are translucent, about 2-3 minutes.
- Add mixed vegetables to the skillet and cook until they are tender yet crisp, about 3-4 minutes.
- Push the vegetables to one side of the skillet and pour the beaten eggs into the other side. Let them cook undisturbed for a minute or until they start to set, then scramble them until cooked through.
- Mix the scrambled eggs with the vegetables in the skillet.

NUTRITIONAL FACTS

- Calories: 180kcal
- Total Fat: 10g
- Total Carbohydrate: 13g
- Dietary Fiber: 5g
- Sugars: 5g
- Protein: 10g

INSTRUCTIONS

- Add the cauliflower rice to the skillet, stirring well to combine with the vegetables and eggs.
- Drizzle soy sauce and sesame oil over the cauliflower rice mixture. Stir well to evenly distribute the flavors.
- If using, add cooked chicken, shrimp, or tofu to the skillet and stir until heated through.
- Season with salt and pepper to taste.
- Garnish with chopped green onions and sesame seeds if desired. Serve hot.

GRILLED PORTOBELLO MUSHROOMS

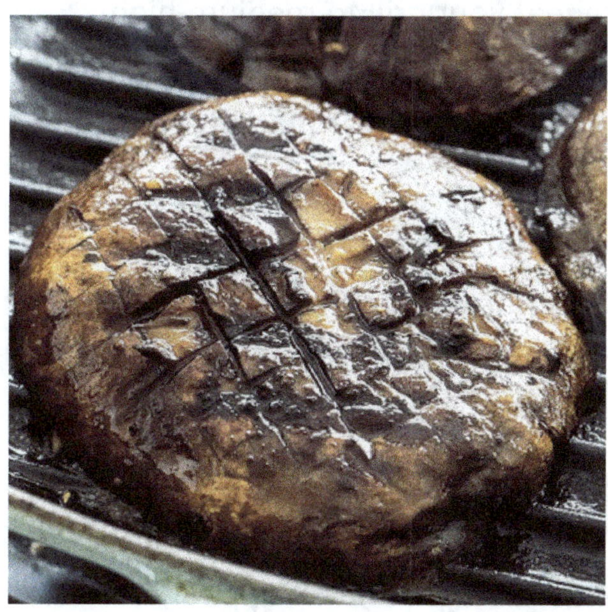

Preparation: 15 minutes

Marinating: 30 minutes

Grilling: 10 minutes

Serving Size: 4

INSTRUCTIONS

- Clean the Portobello mushrooms by wiping them with a damp cloth. Remove the stems and gently scrape out the gills using a spoon. This will create more space for the marinade and prevent excess moisture during grilling.

- In a small bowl, whisk together minced garlic, balsamic vinegar, olive oil, dried thyme, dried oregano, salt, and pepper. Place the cleaned mushrooms in a shallow dish or resealable plastic bag and pour the marinade over them. Ensure each mushroom is well coated. Marinate in the refrigerator for at least 30 minutes, turning occasionally to ensure even marination.

INGREDIENTS

- 4 large portobello mushrooms
- 2 cloves garlic, minced
- 2 tablespoons balsamic vinegar
- 2 tablespoons olive oil
- 1 teaspoon dried thyme
- 1 teaspoon dried oregano
- Salt and pepper to taste
- Fresh parsley for garnish (optional)

NUTRITIONAL FACTS

- Calories: 90 kcal
- Total Fat: 7g
- Saturated Fat: 1g
- Trans Fat: 0g
- Cholesterol: 0mg
- Sodium: 150mg
- Total Carbohydrates: 5g
- Dietary Fiber: 2g
- Sugars: 2g
- Protein: 2g

INSTRUCTIONS

- Preheat your grill to medium-high heat. If using a charcoal grill, ensure the coals are ashed over and spread evenly.
- Once marinated, remove the mushrooms from the marinade and shake off any excess. Place them on the preheated grill, gill side down. Grill for about 4-5 minutes on each side, or until the mushrooms are tender and grill marks appear.
- Transfer the grilled mushrooms to a serving plate. Garnish with fresh parsley if desired. Serve hot as a side dish or as a main course with a side salad or grilled vegetables.

AIR POPPED POPCORN

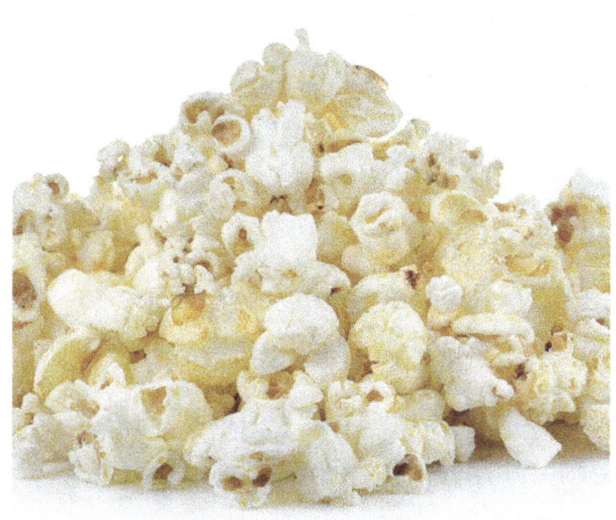

Popping Time: 5 Mins

Serving Size: 3

INGREDIENTS

- 1/4 cup popcorn kernels
- 1/4 teaspoon sea salt (optional)
- 1 teaspoon nutritional yeast (optional, for a cheesy flavor)
- Olive oil spray (optional, for light coating)

NUTRITIONAL FACTS

- Calories: 55 kcal
- Protein: 2g
- Carbohydrates: 12g
- Dietary Fiber: 2g
- Sugars: 0g
- Fat: 0.5g

INSTRUCTIONS

- Set up your air popper according to the manufacturer's instructions.
- Measure out 1/4 cup of popcorn kernels.
- Pour the kernels into the air popper and turn it on. Place a large bowl under the chute to catch the popped popcorn.
- Once the popping slows down to about 2-3 seconds between pops, turn off the popper.
- Lightly spray the popcorn with olive oil if you desire a bit of added flavor and to help seasonings stick.
- Sprinkle sea salt and nutritional yeast over the popcorn. Toss well to evenly distribute the seasoning.

CHICKEN AND VEGGIE KEBABS

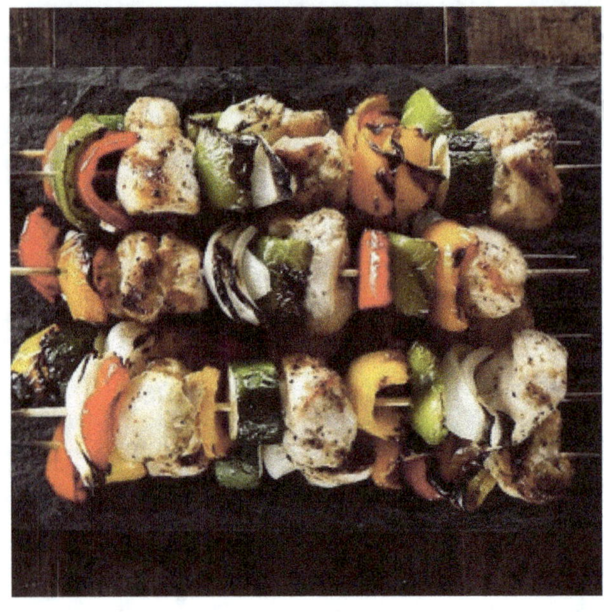

Cook Time: 25 Mins

Serving Size: 4

INGREDIENTS

- 2 boneless, skinless chicken breasts, cut into chunks
- 1 red bell pepper, cut into chunks
- 1 yellow bell pepper, cut into chunks
- 1 red onion, cut into chunks
- 8 cherry tomatoes
- 8 small mushrooms
- 2 tablespoons olive oil
- 2 cloves garlic, minced
- 1 teaspoon paprika
- 1 teaspoon cumin
- Salt and pepper to taste
- Wooden skewers, soaked in water for 30 minutes

INSTRUCTIONS

- In a bowl, combine olive oil, minced garlic, paprika, cumin, salt, and pepper. Add chicken chunks and coat them evenly. Let it marinate for at least 15 minutes.
- Preheat your grill or grill pan over medium-high heat.
- Thread the marinated chicken, bell peppers, onion, cherry tomatoes, and mushrooms onto the soaked wooden skewers, alternating between ingredients.
- Place the kebabs on the preheated grill and cook for about 10-12 minutes, turning occasionally, until the chicken is cooked through and the vegetables are tender and slightly charred.
- Once cooked, remove the kebabs from the grill and let them rest for a few minutes before serving.

NUTRITIONAL FACTS

- Calories: 250 kcal | Protein: 25g | Carbohydrates: 10g
- Fat: 12g | Fiber: 3g | Sugar: 5g

SALMON AND SPINACH SALAD

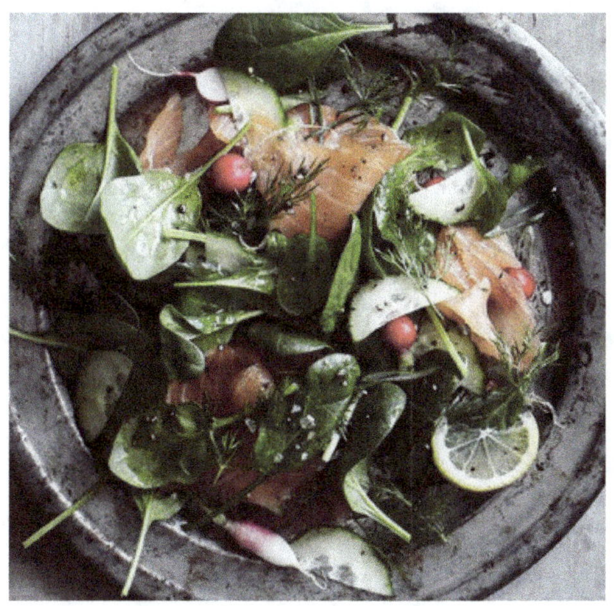

Cook Time: 10 Mins

Serving Size: 2

INGREDIENTS

- 2 salmon fillets (6 oz each)
- 4 cups fresh spinach leaves
- 1 cup cherry tomatoes, halved
- 1/2 cucumber, thinly sliced
- 1/4 red onion, thinly sliced
- 1 avocado, diced
- 2 tablespoons olive oil
- 1 tablespoon lemon juice
- 1 teaspoon Dijon mustard
- Salt and pepper to taste
- Optional: sesame seeds for garnish

NUTRITIONAL FACTS

- Calories: 450kcal | Protein: 30g
- Carbohydrates: 15g
- Fat: 30g | Fiber: 8g | Sugar: 5g

INSTRUCTIONS

- Preheat oven to 400°F (200°C).
- Season the salmon fillets with salt and pepper.
- Place salmon fillets on a baking sheet lined with parchment paper.
- Bake for 10-12 minutes or until salmon is cooked through and flakes easily with a fork.
- In a large mixing bowl, combine spinach, cherry tomatoes, cucumber, red onion, and avocado.
- In a small bowl, whisk together olive oil, lemon juice, Dijon mustard, salt, and pepper to make the dressing.
- Pour the dressing over the salad and toss until well combined.
- Divide the salad onto plates and top with baked salmon fillets.
- Garnish with sesame seeds if desired.
- Serve and enjoy!

IMPORTANCE OF CONSISTENCY

Consistency is key for endomorphs (and for anyone pursuing fitness goals). Without consistency, it's challenging to see meaningful progress. Here's why consistency matters:

- **Progress Tracking:** Consistent exercise allows endomorphs to track their progress accurately. Whether it's weight loss, muscle gain, or improved endurance, consistency makes it easier to measure results over time.

- **Habit Formation:** Regular exercise helps establish a habit. Once exercise becomes a routine part of daily life, it's easier to stick to it long-term.

- **Metabolic Adaptation:** Consistent exercise helps the body adapt and become more efficient at burning calories and building muscle. Over time, this leads to better metabolic health and improved body composition.

- **Mental Benefits:** Exercise is not only beneficial for physical health but also for mental well-being. Consistent physical activity can reduce stress, anxiety, and depression, leading to a better overall quality of life.

- **Long-Term Sustainability:** Consistency fosters a sustainable approach to fitness. Rather than relying on short-term fixes or crash diets, consistent exercise promotes long-term health and fitness goals.

BALANCING CARDIO AND STRENGTH TRAINING

Balancing cardiovascular exercise with strength training is essential for endomorphs to achieve optimal results. Here's how to strike the right balance:

- **Prioritize Strength Training:** While cardiovascular exercise is important for calorie burning, endomorphs should prioritize strength training to build lean muscle mass. Muscle tissue burns more calories at rest than fat tissue, contributing to a higher metabolism.
- **Include Both in Your Routine:** Aim for a mix of cardiovascular exercise and strength training throughout the week. This could involve alternating days for each type of workout or incorporating both into a single session.
- **Customize Intensity:** The intensity of cardiovascular and strength workouts can be customized based on individual fitness levels and goals. High-intensity interval training (HIIT) can be particularly effective for combining cardio and strength benefits in one session.
- **Listen to Your Body:** Pay attention to how your body responds to different types of exercise. Some endomorphs may find they need more recovery time between intense cardio sessions, while others may thrive on a higher frequency of strength training.
- **Periodization:** Periodizing your training program by alternating between phases of higher cardio focus and higher strength focus can prevent plateaus and promote continuous progress.

LIST OF EXERCISES

The key for endomorphs is a combination of cardiovascular exercise to burn fat and strength training to build and maintain muscle. Here is a list of exercises suitable for endomorphs along with instructions on how to perform them:

CARDIOVASCULAR EXERCISES

1. **Running or Jogging**
   - **How to perform:** Start with a warm-up of brisk walking or light jogging for 5-10 minutes. Then, increase your speed to a comfortable running pace. Maintain good posture, keeping your back straight and your shoulders relaxed. Aim to run for at least 20-30 minutes.

2. **Cycling**
   - **How to perform:** Use a stationary bike or a regular bicycle. Begin with a warm-up at a low resistance for 5-10 minutes. Increase the resistance or speed gradually. Maintain a steady pace for 30-45 minutes.

3. **Swimming**
   - **How to perform:** Start with a few minutes of easy swimming to warm up. Choose a stroke that you are comfortable with, such as freestyle or breaststroke. Swim continuously for 20-30 minutes, taking breaks if needed.

4. **High-Intensity Interval Training (HIIT)**
   - **How to perform:** Alternate between short bursts of intense activity (e.g., sprinting for 30 seconds) and periods of lower intensity (e.g., walking for 1 minute). Repeat for 20-30 minutes.

STRENGTH TRAINING EXERCISES

1. **Squats**
   - **How to perform:** Stand with your feet shoulder-width apart. Lower your body as if you are sitting in a chair, keeping your back straight and knees over your toes. Go as low as you can without losing form, then return to the starting position. Do 3 sets of 12-15 reps.

2. **Deadlifts**
   - **How to perform:** Stand with feet hip-width apart. Bend at your hips and knees to grab a barbell with an overhand grip. Keep your back straight and lift the barbell by straightening your hips and knees. Lower the bar back to the ground. Do 3 sets of 10-12 reps.

3. **Push-Ups**
   - **How to perform:** Start in a plank position with hands slightly wider than shoulder-width apart. Lower your body until your chest nearly touches the floor, keeping your elbows at a 45-degree angle. Push back up to the starting position. Do 3 sets of 10-15 reps.

4. **Pull-Ups**
   - **How to perform:** Grab a pull-up bar with an overhand grip, hands shoulder-width apart. Pull your body up until your chin is above the bar. Lower back down to the starting position. If you can't do a full pull-up, use an assisted pull-up machine or resistance bands. Do 3 sets of as many reps as possible.

5. **Plank**
   - **How to perform:** Lie face down on the floor. Lift your body up on your toes and forearms, keeping your body in a straight line from head to heels. Hold this position for as long as possible, aiming for at least 30 seconds. Do 3 sets.

FLEXIBILITY AND MOBILITY EXERCISES

1. **Yoga**
   - **How to perform:** Follow a yoga routine that includes poses like Downward Dog, Warrior Poses, and Child's Pose. Focus on breathing and holding each pose for several breaths. Aim for a 20-30 minute session.
2. **Dynamic Stretching**
   - **How to perform:** Perform movements that take your muscles through their full range of motion, such as leg swings, arm circles, and lunges with a twist. Do this as part of your warm-up for 5-10 minutes.

TIPS FOR SUCCESS

- **Consistency:** Regular exercise is key for endomorphs. Aim for at least 150 minutes of moderate-intensity or 75 minutes of high-intensity exercise each week.
- **Diet:** Complement your exercise routine with a balanced diet rich in whole foods, lean proteins, and plenty of vegetables. Control portion sizes to manage caloric intake.
- **Rest:** Ensure you get enough rest and recovery. Aim for 7-9 hours of sleep per night and include rest days in your exercise routine.

By combining these exercises with a healthy diet and adequate rest, endomorphs can effectively manage their weight and improve their overall fitness.

NOTE:

NOTE:

NOTE:

www.ingramcontent.com/pod-product-compliance
Lightning Source LLC
Chambersburg PA
CBHW081807250726
48653CB00010B/3820